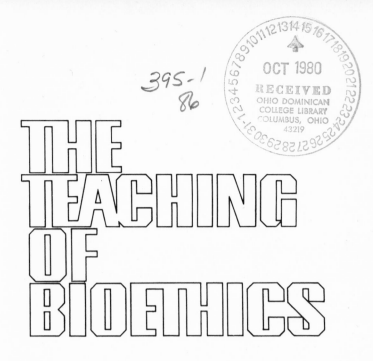

THE TEACHING OF BIOETHICS

Report of the Commission on the Teaching of Bioethics

THE HASTINGS CENTER
Institute of Society, Ethics and the Life Sciences

This report was coordinated by the Education Program of the Institute of Society, Ethics and the Life Sciences under a grant from the Robert Wood Johnson Foundation.

174.2
C 734 I
1976

Institute of Society, Ethics and the Life Sciences
360 Broadway
Hastings-on-Hudson, New York 10706

Library of Congress Cataloging in Publication Data

Commission on the Teaching of Bioethics.
  The teaching of bioethics.

  Bibliography: p.
  1. Bioethics—Study and teaching.   I.   Title.
QH332.C65   1976   174' .2'071   76-44214
ISBN 0-916558-00-2

Printed in the United States of America

CONTENTS

Pub 1.95

COMMISSION MEMBERS

Daniel Callahan, Ph.D., Director, Institute of Society, Ethics and the Life Sciences, Hastings-on-Hudson, New York.

Charles M. Culver, M.D., Ph.D., Associate Professor, Department of Psychiatry, Dartmouth Medical School, Hanover, New Hampshire.

Albert R. Jonsen, Ph.D., Associate Professor of Bioethics, Departments of Medicine and Pediatrics, School of Medicine, University of California at San Francisco.

Ruth Kolman, M.S., teacher, Princeton Day School, Princeton, N.J.

Karen Lebacqz, Ph.D., Assistant Professor of Christian Ethics and Co-director, Joint Program in Bioethics, Pacific School of Religion, Berkeley, California.

Jane A. Raible, D.Min. candidate, Executive Director of the Northwest Institute of Ethics and the Life Sciences, Seattle, Washington.

David H. Smith, Ph.D., Associate Professor and Chairman, Department of Religious Studies, Indiana University, Bloomington.

Robert M. Veatch, Ph.D., Senior Associate, Institute of Society, Ethics and the Life Sciences, Hastings-on-Hudson, New York.

LeRoy Walters, Ph.D., Director of the Center for Bioethics of the Joseph and Rose Kennedy Institute for the Study of Human Reproduction and Bioethics, Georgetown University, Washington, D.C.

PREFACE

In the last decade medical and biological ethics has grown from a rather esoteric teaching enterprise to a major phenomenon. Courses are now offered not only in medical schools and seminaries, but also in undergraduate departments of philosophy, religion, sociology, and biology as well as in grade schools and senior citizen adult education programs. Since its founding in 1969, the Institute of Society, Ethics and the Life Sciences has been committed to assisting universities, medical and professional schools in the development of programs designed to integrate a consideration of ethical problems into the formal education process as well as to supporting programs aimed at reaching the general public. The Institute began its educational involvement with a two-year project to develop a medical ethics teaching program at Columbia University's College of Physicians and Surgeons. It has also been involved in teaching programs in colleges and universities, adult education programs, law schools, and professional continuing education.

As interest in teaching medical and biological ethics grew, we thought several innovations were necessary in order to continue to provide support and service. In 1972 we began a series of medical ethics workshops designed for beginning teachers in this field. As of the summer of 1976, we have had over 500 participants. We also began a reading reprint series for classroom use, which provides easy access to over one hundred articles from widely divergent sources. Additionally, we thought that it was time to step back and examine the rapid growth and possible future of this teaching field. We had been asked to advise foundations in deciding whether a relatively wealthy medical school or a struggling undergraduate philosophy department ought to get limited funds to start a medical ethics teaching program. We had been asked by administrators whether physicians or philos-

v

ophers ought to be doing the teaching in a medical school and what institutional settings had proved most effective as the locus of medical ethics teaching. We had been asked whether courses should be organized around issues (such as euthanasia and abortion) or around themes (such as freedom and truth-telling). We had been asked whether we need more basic texts and whether audiovisual materials are in adequate supply.

This report is an attempt to aid teachers, school administrators, and officials from public agencies and foundations who are making those and other decisions about the establishment of medical ethics teaching programs.

It is the product of a Commission on the Teaching of Bioethics established in 1973 to get a broader perspective on the discipline's evolution. The Commission's members had taught medical ethics at widely different levels (many at more than one) from grade school to graduate academic and professional school teaching. They had disciplinary backgrounds in medicine, the humanities, and the social sciences. All had sufficient experience to see medical and biological ethics teaching in some perspective.

We are aware of other historical examples of commissions established to examine the evolution of a new field. We are further aware of a frequent pattern: to use such a commission to legitimate the field, to establish standards for licensure, and to develop ways of excluding "unqualified practitioners." We are concerned about all of these issues, but, conscious of that history and committed to the belief that medical and biological ethics is necessarily an interdisciplinary enterprise, we have resisted proposals to establish a formal professional organization, certification, and the other equipment of a professional group. While we do make some strong recommendations about training and teaching standards, the needs of the field, and the areas which ought to receive more attention, it is with the recognition that medical and biological ethics is very interdisciplinary and very young, at least in its present manifestation.

One of the problems of the evolution of teaching in this area has been the proliferation of names of the field itself. Originally we tended to talk about teaching "medical ethics," but that was taken by some to exclude ethical problems in biology such as basic research in genetics. On the other hand, the term "biological ethics" might not adequately capture the medical issues that have been a central concern. The phrase "medical and biological ethics" covers both areas, but is cumbersome. Recently the short term "bioethics" has been used. It has its problems, too. It might not adequately capture the medical dimensions. It might imply to some that we are dealing with a field independent of ethics as a parent discipline. Nevertheless, for convenience we have adopted "bioethics" as an inclusive label for our area of concern. By it we mean the range of issues that could also be called "medical and biological ethics."

We are grateful to the Robert Wood Johnson Foundation for supporting the Commission through most of its work, and to the Rockefeller Brothers Fund, the Hazen Foundation, and the National Endowment for the Humanities for supporting the related work of the Institute's Education Program.

—Robert M. Veatch
Senior Associate and
Director, Education Programs
Institute of Society, Ethics
and the Life Sciences

PART ONE

Bioethics: Its Nature and Future

At least since the time of Hippocrates people have recognized that morality has a central place in the practice of medicine. Moral codes and discussion of ethical theory have a long and honored place in both philosophical and medical literature. Yet until very recently, the domain of medical ethics was seen in a relatively narrow focus, primarily physicians' professional obligations to each other and to their patients. It was not until the biological sciences rapidly rose to prominence in the twentieth century that the scope of medical ethics expanded to include the basic biological research upon which clinical practice is scientifically based. While clinical applications of the new biological knowledge grew rapidly in this period, biomedicine became as well a major facet of contemporary life. This development has been marked by an increase in the proportion of the Gross National Product going to medical research and treatment, massive governmental support of biomedical research, a phenomenal growth in the drug and other medically related industries, and a very rapid increase in the cost and complexity of medical care.

At the same time, broad social and cultural changes have affected medical structures and decision making. Human rights and individual autonomy have become dominant political themes. Authoritarian and hierarchical decision making has, at least in many sectors, yielded to pluralism and personal freedom of choice. On the other hand, there has been increasing bureau-

1

cratization and development of complex social institutions to deal with public problems. The complex medical care system is an example.

Accompanying these social and technological changes, and intimately related to them both as cause and effect, is our increasing social concern with personal and environmental health. The formerly simple definitions of familiar terms, such as "health," "sickness," "illness," "disability," and the like, are now laden with conceptual and practical problems. Furthermore, this new awareness has forced an examination of the relative value of health in relationship to, and often in competition with, other social goods (education, national security, and urban life, for example).

Taken together, these developments have resulted in a significantly different societal role for medical research and clinical application, a shift in the place and function of the physician, and a change in the relative importance of biomedicine compared with other areas of political and social life. They have been paralleled by a whole range of new and unprecedented moral dilemmas in biomedicine. Some bear on the proper use of new medical powers to intervene in human procreation, to modify behavior, and to influence the course of death. Others have focused on medicine's goals, concepts of health and illness, and the relation between bodily welfare and those other goods which humans seek. Still other dilemmas have arisen because of the changes in doctor-patient relationships occasioned by high technology and increased specialization, by problems inherent in the delivery of mass medical care, and by a growing uncertainty about the appropriate role of medicine in areas once thought beyond its scope.

Biomedicine is undergoing a rapid transformation, both in terms of its perceived goals and the appropriate means to achieve them. When any major social institution goes through a period of transformation, ethical questions come to the fore. Social and technological change force a reexamination of traditional values, a fresh look at traditional goals, a recognition of wider potential ones, and a new critique of the relationship between ends and means.

What Is Bioethics?

The field of bioethics has been one important reponse to the emergence of critical value and ethical issues. The term "bioethics" is itself a neologism, denoting a concern not simply with medical ethics but, more broadly, with the full range of ethical issues arising from advances in medicine and biology. Thus it encompasses much of concern to traditional medical ethics, but includes a great deal more as well. To speak, however, of a "field of bioethics" is perhaps to endow the widespread interest in the subject with somewhat more reality than the current situation warrants. If by a "field" is meant a well-demarcated area of research and teaching, with recognized canons and standards, then bioethics has not yet achieved that status. But if it is taken to mean a general area of concern, marked by publications and courses, interest and debate, then bioethics surely qualifies.

The term "bioethics" implies a focus on those normative questions that have traditionally been discussed in the discipline of ethics. Three major normative questions are raised in ethics. First, what kinds of actions are morally right? Second, what kinds of character are morally praiseworthy? And third, what states of affairs are most worthwhile? Therefore, bioethics can be seen as an attempt to ask these kinds of questions as they arise in the context of biomedical research and practice.

Those working and teaching in the field need to grasp concepts of normative ethics that have been developed in philosophy and theology over the centuries. No serious grappling with practical issues of medicine and biology can avoid an attempt to understand, articulate, and criticize those broad ethical principles which set the stage for the specific rules of conduct meant to govern human behavior in specific contexts. As one attempts to apply ethics to certain biomedical areas, the meaning and application of such principles as "do no harm" and "respect the sanctity of life" are no longer clear. Other questions that arise include how ethical principles can conflict with each other, what specific rules of conduct should be, and whether those rules should be binding in every circumstance. General and specific questions of normative ethics cannot be avoided and there are better and worse ways of approaching them. But is it enough to limit bioethics to such an examination?

For a number of reasons we believe it would be a mistake to limit bioethics only to philosophical or theological methods, however critical and central these may be. Bioethics has arisen as an interdisciplinary field, one of the few where cooperation and discourse across the usual boundaries have been both intense and fruitful. It has attracted people working in theology, philosophy, law, and social sciences, life sciences, and various branches of the humanities. These disciplines all tend to have characteristic interests, methodologies, and predilections which color their understanding. No one field has been able to claim a monopoly on the issues, and many fields have simultaneously felt the impact of the problems. The areas of genetic counseling, psychosurgery, or treatment of dying patients raise economic, legal, social, and cultural as well as philosophical and theological questions. Moreover, from a systematic point of view, the difficulty and pervasiveness of the issues invites, even if it does not make easy, the adoption of a broad-ranging point of view. This is particularly the case when matters of public policy—which must, in our society, take account of ethical, constitutional, and legislative values and norms—are at stake.

This is *not* to say that ethics can be reduced to problems of law, or problems of law to issues of ethics; or that moral norms can be derived from attitudes and values measured in sociological studies; or that ethics cannot be separated from religion, or religion from ethics. That remains an open question. But it is to say that the way in which values are shaped and norms developed is an enormously complex process which cannot neatly be parceled out among standard disciplines and fields. Since many of the most critical issues in bioethics turn not simply on how an individual should make up his or her mind, or on how specific rules of behavior should be framed, but, more importantly, on whole patterns of private, public, governmental and institutional life, multiple perspectives are both necessary and productive.

Yet to assert the value of interdisciplinary work in the field of bioethics (that is, to deny that the field should be reduced to the methods and perspectives of philosophy or theology) by no means solves the pedagogical problem of establishing appropriate tasks and roles for the varied disciplines making up the field. Normative questions are the point of confluence: what individuals *ought* to do (or may be wise to do); how legislation *ought* to be framed and policy established. Various disciplines can make different contributions to the resolution of these questions. Metaethics (the examination of modes of ethical argumentation and justification) and empirical social sciences (the description of the actual practices of individuals and institutions) are very different kinds of activities; nonetheless both can contribute usefully to public discussion.

While the exact relationship between normative ethics and other disciplines is a matter of debate, certain of its general features can be discussed. Medicine and the social, behavioral, and biological sciences provide descriptive and predictive methods and information which set the context for ethical reflection. Ethics, on the other hand, provides the logic of moral arguments as well as the analysis of moral principles and values; both help to understand why a moral problem arises in a certain situation and what the various moral options are for its resolution. We are convinced that bioethics must move beyond descriptive study to critical investigation of alternative norms, goals, and personal and social ideals.

The purpose of this report is to confront one important range of questions posed by the emergence—haphazard as it is intense—of bioethics. Many of those questions, in various forms, center on the problem of education. Who should receive an education in bioethics? What should such an education include? Who should teach bioethics? In what way should bioethics be taught? What are the relative priorities in the levels of teaching of bioethics? What are the goals of courses in bioethics? These questions arise because a great and growing number of courses and teaching programs on ethical problems in medicine and biology are being offered throughout the country. But there is no uniformity in how the problems are defined, or in how such courses are taught. Given such diversity, many are pressed to ask how such courses should be organized and taught; still others, with institutional responsibilities, must determine which should receive money and support. The fact that courses are now offered from the high school level through undergraduate and professional education to the postprofessional itself makes agreement on the nature and quality of such teaching difficult.

Goals of Bioethics Teaching

What should be the goals of the teaching of bioethics? At least four general goals can be posited, although there will be differences in emphasis at different educational levels and settings.

1. *Identifying and defining moral issues*

First, the teaching of bioethics should help students identify moral issues in a biomedical context and understand what it means for something to be a moral issue. Often the evaluative dimension of biomedical decisions is buried and thus difficult to recognize. For example, it is presumed without question that the dying cancer patient must have surgery or that the person in chronic renal failure needs a kidney transplant. Both seem, at first, to be technical problems with technical solutions. While it may be a medical fact that their chances of survival for a certain period will increase, it is not a fact that they must have these procedures. Rather it is an evaluation—implicit or explicit—of the alternatives. Even if it is an evaluation, however, students of bioethics should also learn to differentiate moral issues from those of personal or group taste. One of the basic purposes of teaching of ethics is to clarify the meaning of terms such as "moral" and "ethical," as well as prescriptive words such as "should," "ought," and "must." The student should know how the meanings of these terms vary and what the differences are between using them in a moral sense and in other senses.

An ability to distinguish facts from values and ethical from other kinds of evaluations will help to clarify the different roles in the decision-making process. The result may be the realization by some who do not think that they should have a role in the decision-making process that they do have such a role. Or, those who assume they alone have a decision-making role may recognize the appropriate role of others.

2. Developing strategies and analyzing moral problems

Once one has learned to recognize a moral problem, what then? A second goal of bioethics teaching should be to develop strategies for analyzing moral problems. Moral principles, rules, and rights provide a framework. Thus, a course in bioethics may have as one of its goals the explicit examination of alternative systems of principles, rules, and rights, or it may compare and contrast the use of principles, rules, and rights as an approach to moral problems with a direct examination of situations to intuit what is right or wrong. Finally, developing any strategy for analyzing moral problems will require thinking about what one should do when principles, rules, rights, or intuitions about situations conflict.

If one learns that deciding for or against cancer surgery requires ethical and other value determinations, as well as considerations of fact, one then might want to know what principles or guidelines are available. One principle is that the physicians should always do what they think will benefit their patients. Another is that they should protect patient freedom and thus not treat without consent. Another rule primary to some is that life ought to be preserved. Quite clearly these principles and rules can conflict. One ordering principle might be that when rules conflict one should always take precedence (such as preserving life, promoting happiness or preserving freedom). Another is that the conflicting principles should be balanced. One goal of bioethics courses may be to further the systematic study of such principles and plans for resolving conflict. A bioethics course might become a context for learning ethical theory or it might examine these questions of principle in order to facilitate a third goal.

3. Relating moral principles to specific issues and cases

A third goal of the teaching of bioethics is to assist individuals and institutions in resolving moral conflicts that are related to specific issues and cases. This requires an ability to see the implications of both moral principles and the ways in which conflicting principles may be resolved. It also requires an ability to envision and articulate the role of moral principles in the development of codes of behavior and practice, of decision-making procedures, and of the relationship among established attitudes, preferences, and latent assumptions.

In the case of the cancer patient who must choose whether or not to have surgery, it is not enough to recognize that there are ethical and other evaluative considerations at stake. It is also not enough to know which principles might apply and which procedures for conflict resolution are most appropriate. In the end the decision makers must work their way through to a conclusion. The patient must choose either for or against the surgery. The physician must choose whether to accept that patient's decision or to withdraw from the case on grounds of conscience.

4. *Training a group for careers in bioethics*

Finally, the fourth goal of some bioethics courses should be to train those people who plan careers in bioethics. These include teachers of bioethics courses, staff members of research institutes, and occasionally lawyers, clergy, and physicians who may make the field of bioethics their primary vocation. Some—but certainly not all—teaching programs will have the training of a cadre of bioethicists as a major objective.

Each of these four goals is important, although different courses in different disciplines and at different levels of teaching emphasize them in quite different ways. The field itself would not have developed—nor developed with such a special sense of urgency—had not problems arisen in all four areas. Furthermore, within a particular level learning to recognize the ethical issue may be the primary task in some instances while in others gaining experience in working the moral problem through to a solution will be important. Learning to recognize the moral problem will be crucial even though the student may not be the major decision maker in a particular case. In fact, one of the most important things to learn may be when not to work through the problem to an answer but to defer to others. On the other hand, when the student will be directly responsible for making a decision, then learning to recognize the problem as a moral one is only the first step. Just what constitutes an "ethical" issue and an appropriate sound method of analyzing moral principles? How ought we to go about unearthing the contents and ramifications of principles, or devising ways in which intense policy conflicts that rest on latent or manifest moral disagreement can be resolved? A recognition that one cannot begin to make rational decisions in medicine and biology without a vigorous effort to bring ethical issues to the surface, to develop analytic tools to grapple with them, and to develop techniques for resolving moral issues, is the basis upon which the teaching of bioethics must be built.

While there are many valid purposes for teaching bioethics, one purpose is sometimes cited that we consider to be dubious: that teaching bioethics will make the student more humane or humanitarian. Although bioethics lies within the broad area of the humanities, there is an important difference between the humanities as a discipline and humanitarianism. The special purpose of bioethics teaching should not be to increase humanitarianism. If such an increase results at all it derives more generally from the educational experience and the role models for life styles and value perspectives that students see in their teachers and friends. Presumably every teacher hopes that students will leave a course changed in their ability to think, reason, or act—and this applies also to courses in the humanities, including bioethics, but bioethics is in no way unique in this hope.

Patterns of Bioethics Teaching

As a teaching field, bioethics has displayed some patterns of development and posed some problems. Among the questions frequently asked are: what format should be used for teaching, how should the curriculum be organized, who should teach bioethics, how should it be structured administratively, what ought to be the priorities?

1. *What format should be used for teaching?*

Many different formats have been used for bioethics teaching. Traditional lectures and seminars are among the obvious, but other methods have been used as well. In clinical settings, such as hospitals, case presentations and grand rounds have become an important teaching vehicle. Individual instruction through tutorials or intensive internships has been used. Many schools have introduced bioethics through noncredit lecture series or conferences. Several institutions have successfully organized students into teams which examine the medical, ethical, and legal dimensions of an emerging biomedical area and recommend an appropriate public policy.

Clearly, different formats serve different purposes; each is useful under certain conditions. Two general conclusions can be made, however. First, a lecture course which precludes direct student participation in the struggle with ideas is inadequate. While guest lecture series are sometimes useful to stimulate student or faculty interest, they should be used to lead to something with greater depth and integration. Second, case presentations or grand rounds, while seemingly very relevant, are always in danger of avoiding more systematic reflection. When possible, these should always be coordinated with opportunities for more systematic thinking.

2. *How should the curriculum be organized?*

Courses have been structured in at least three different ways: *topical*, *thematic*, or *methodic*. A topical course deals with a series of topics of current interest in bioethics. Its syllabus consists of an index listing such subjects as "genetic counseling," "transplantation and dialysis," and "psychosurgery." An effort is made to expose the relevant moral issues under each topic. A thematic course touches these same topics but does so under explicit overall themes, such as truth-telling, confidentiality, freedom, consent, "medical paternalism," and "justice and health care." Here the topics are illustrative or exemplary for analysis of a theme. Finally, a methodic course uses topics or themes but is principally interested in conveying an analytic method; e.g., the method of ethical analysis, stressing utilitarian or deontological modes of ethical reasoning, or socio-ethical analyses, stressing critical perception of the values of institutions, social structures, and behavior.

Our view of bioethics suggests that the introductory course content should be primarily thematic. Purely topical presentations tend to become overly particularistic and fractured and to make more difficult an appreciation of the recurring themes.

3. Who should teach bioethics courses?

One common pattern of bioethics teaching, particularly at the undergraduate level and in medical schools, has been team-teaching. The guiding assumption has frequently been that bioethics is best understood from at least two perspectives: the scientific or clinical, and the general and theoretical (e.g., philosophical). Advocates say this method balances very concrete cases and problems with those general principles that transcend specific issues. Another pattern has been to teach from a single disciplinary perspective such as that of philosophy or religion. Such courses, frequently taught by one person (often with visiting lecturers), attempt to develop a coherent and systematic framework for analyzing biomedical problems. Still another pattern has been a broadly interdisciplinary course, which draws from three or more disciplines to study different ways of approaching issues.

However the course is taught, the teaching staff must have competence in both ethics and the biomedical sciences. An ideal teacher would have professional competence in both ethics and biology or medicine. But the problems inherent in such highly specialized dual training, combined with the probable difficulty of maintaining full professional standing either as ethicist or as scientist/clinician, make such a teacher unusual. An alternative is for teachers to be competent professionals in one area with "competent amateur" standing in the other. A team of two such individuals is, in our opinion, the best possible combination in institutional settings where at least two staff appointments can be made. These various patterns all have advantages and disadvantages. Local needs, the interests of teachers, and the composition of student bodies can vary so much that it is impossible to assert some ideal pattern.

4. *How should bioethics be structured administratively?*

As patterns of teaching vary, so do administrative patterns. Sometimes bioethics courses are sponsored by science departments. In other instances, departments of philosophy or religion provide the administrative framework. In the health sciences, clinical departments including medicine, pediatrics, psychiatry, and family medicine, have housed bioethics teaching.

Another administrative pattern is based on the interdisciplinary character of bioethics. Some courses are cosponsored, for instance, by philosophy and biology departments. Others are sponsored by interdisciplinary programs of science and society, the humanities, or public policy. Additionally, some people advocate new departments of bioethics or interdisciplinary programs. This structure is especially promising when officially designated representatives from the relevant existing departments participate. It avoids the fragmentation of department sponsorship and still uses the resources of existing departments.

It is often critical to establish an administratively identifiable program with its own funding and faculty appointments so that at least some teachers see themselves and are seen primarily as bioethics teachers. If any ideal is to be asserted, it would be the value of a full program in bioethics, that is, a range of integrated courses, some designed for those just beginning study of the field, others for those at a more advanced level; or some focusing on a broad range of problems, with others focusing in more depth on a single problem. The field itself is so rich and complex that no single course can do it full justice; and like any other field, there should be provision for different interests and degrees of preparation.

5. *What ought to be our priorities?*

At the moment few schools are in a position to develop full programs, because of scarce funds and inadequately trained staff. For some time to come, the emphasis will be on individual courses within particular departments. Many school and university authorities, as well as funding agencies, will inevitably have to determine the relative priorities to be given different possibilities at different levels of education. While this problem will be addressed directly in Part Three of this report, one general comment is in order at this point.

The most important need at the moment is for programs and courses of high quality. The field is too new and too tentative to tolerate poor courses; in many places, students will get one and only one systematic introduction to the problems, with little chance for a second exposure. In those places a poor course would be worse than no course at all. Moreover, as administrations are forced to evaluate competing demands for different kinds of courses and programs, it is vital that they not witness poor courses or experiments. The importance of the subject matter and its implications for future lives and public policy underscores even more the need for quality and seriousness.

This report is designed to assist those teaching courses or planning to do so, those organizing programs, and those who must allocate funds or resources to the field of bioethics. Given the great diversity of settings in which bioethics can be taught—from elementary schools through graduate and postprofessional programs in bioethics—the focus will be upon the problems and goals at different levels and in different settings. This approach seems preferable to, and potentially more helpful than, a general, abstract approach which would attempt to deal with all levels and settings simultaneously. Each of the sections under Part Two considers the present scope and extent of teaching; goals and instructional objectives; formats for teaching; curriculum organization; qualifications for teaching; future needs and priorities within specific settings; and problems of funding and personnel. While not all of these issues will be treated with an equal emphasis in each subsection, they comprise the range of important problems which we believe arise when courses and programs are established. Part Three of the report addresses the question of relative priorities among different levels of teaching.

PART TWO

The Scope of
Bioethics Teaching

A. ELEMENTARY AND SECONDARY SCHOOLS*

I. Existing Programs

Sometimes people do not realize that bioethics education does in fact start early in the educational process—in elementary and secondary schools. While few programs are labeled "bioethics," the topics and behavioral objectives that are central to good bioethics teaching are being used in such curriculum areas as value clarification, human development, social awareness, historical perspectives, and religion. Sometimes, particularly in the upper grades, these efforts are conscious attempts to introduce students to the field. More often, however, a teacher who has never heard of the term "bioethics" intuitively attempts to create a classroom atmosphere in which children can learn about and prepare for some of the experiences that they will meet in life.

There is a growing feeling that even preschool children must learn about death as well as birth, and be able to express both happy and sad feelings. One response is that of the nursery school teacher who skillfully guided one of her four-year-old

*This section of the report was written primarily by Ruth Kolman who teaches at the Princeton Day School, Princeton, N.J.

students into an explanation of why she was unusually sad that day. After a certain amount of evasion, the little girl explained to her classmates that her cat had given birth to kittens and had eaten one of them. The discussion turned to death—what is it like, when should it come? Such a nursery school discussion might not fall under the rubric of classical bioethics, but it can begin a continuum and create an atmosphere conducive to the development of an awareness of, and ability to cope with, such complex issues.

In addition to such informal incorporation of sensitive issues into the framework of existing curricula, there are a limited but rapidly growing number of formal courses and course modules explicitly dealing with bioethics. A great many teachers have demonstrated interest in teaching bioethics courses, and undoubtedly will do this, as soon as curriculum formats and resource material become available.

II. Goals

Central to the goals of bioethics teaching is a belief that education should focus on the student's total personal development in addition to mastery of cognitive skills. This expanded educational goal aims at developing sensitivity, self-awareness, confidence, the ability to make rational decisions, and the ability to recognize a moral dilemma.

To develop curricula that will satisfy these goals, the most important factor to recognize in elementary and high school students is their youth. The fact is so obvious that it might very well be overlooked. If that occurred, the key to good teaching would be thrown away: that is, to determine the level of student cognitive and moral development, and to use that determination as a basis on which to build. More simply, it is necessary to understand students' experiences and to develop an awareness of the nature of their social and factual understanding.

When we hear twelve-year-olds cogently discussing the concepts of Mendelian genetics and Darwinian evolution, it is easy to forget the limited set of experiences confronted by these children. Of course, childhood is full of difficulties, frustrations, and emotional conflicts, but these usually do not compare in kind or complexity with the experiences of older students. Medical students come to class straight from their rounds in the wards and their stints in the clinics. Adult education classes often attract people who have had a profound experience that has challenged the foundation of their moral structure. In comparison, in some areas many K-12 students are still beautifully naive.

The teacher who wishes to explore with children the ethical dilemmas that occur in the life cycle should use a two-pronged approach. First, it is necessary to establish an experimental and cognitive base that is primarily geared to expanding knowledge, and upon which open discussion can take place. Second, the teacher must establish an atmosphere of free and honest inquiry. An elementary school teacher might satisfy these goals by maintaining a family of small animals. Students could observe and discuss changes in behavior during various phases of the life cycle. This will include mating, birth, maternal care, growth, successive generations. It will also include mothers eating their less fit young, and the inevitable death of the old and the weak.

In such a situation it is important that teachers treat all parts of the life cycle with the same honesty and frankness. This allows students to express feelings about such things as death, parental behavior control, serious illness, and aging. The birth of a gerbil in a nursery school classroom is often welcomed and thoroughly discussed; the death of the same animal is often glossed over hurriedly. Sometimes teachers even go to great extremes to hide the fact that a classroom pet has died. While attempting to protect their students from unhappiness, these well-meaning, conscientious teachers are maintaining a classroom taboo by not acknowledging death. Instead of protecting the sensibilities of children, these taboos often produce a fear of the unknown and the unspoken. As such they serve to prevent the later development of an ability to approach moral dilemmas rationally.

Bioethics, in whatever form it appears in the curriculum, should be oriented toward helping students recognize and reflect upon moral dilemmas. By carefully choosing course material, students can be forced to focus on value conflicts. A high school history class studying the world food crisis, for example, can be led to confront conflicting views on causes of population growth. A discussion of the possible solutions can touch on dilemma-filled concepts such as human dignity, personhood, individual rights, and group (social) responsibility.

A mathematics teacher can use data collected from HEW or WHO in units on statistics or graphing as a way of involving students in consideration of bioethical issues. Students may find it hard to believe the differences between life expectancy rates for whites and nonwhites in this country, just as they may be astonished at the vital statistics collected from Third World countries.

A modern biology course, because of the topics into which it delves, must include some discussion of conflicting values. Heated discussions begin as soon as students learn about genetic defects. Teachers are forced to make a decision: should they avoid discussion of, say, society's responsibilities for people with genetic anomalies, because the course is already so full of cognitive material that the subject cannot adequately be covered in the time allotted? Or should they take the approach that modern science should not be taught in an ethical vacuum, and therefore set aside time for discussions of conflicting values? If administrators want the latter alternative, they have to find time themselves to encourage, support, and advise such teachers.

Finally, bioethics education should help prepare students to make decisions about their own health. The proliferation of medical technology and medical expertise is capable of drastically changing our concept of humanness, and it is part of the educators' responsibility to enable students to learn whatever might be necessary to cope with the advances of science and medicine. This involves both the learning of factual material and the development of personally appropriate attitudes.

At this level there are at least two categories of important health-related decisions. One is decisions individuals make as consumers of medical care. To this end students should learn about such things as informed consent, patients' bill of rights, commitment procedures, and health care economics. The second category is related to life style. Students are confronted with decisions about their own sexual behavior and the use of tobacco, drugs, and alcohol. In each case they make value-laden decisions, either consciously or inadvertently, and they resolve their own moral dilemmas.

Our schools are not doing enough to help students make responsible decisions. Health education time is still used to teach students how to brush their teeth, rather than to help them confront their own biomedical dilemmas. Even though our teen-age students are on the brink of having to make major decisions, classroom practice tends to avoid the profound issues. Too often students get their best guidance in the least important elements of their life.

III. Teaching Formats

The teaching format will vary depending on the grade level, type of course, and classroom structure. However, any successful format must allow for free and open discussion, so that students can express the most extreme points of view without fear of criticism or ridicule. It is equally important that a body of knowledge be carefully established so that opinions are not based on ignorance. Knowing how to get the facts is an important prerequisite of rational decision making.

Many strategies can be used to stimulate discussion, including audiovisual presentations and visits by professionals such as lawyers, physicians, and medical researchers. Field trips to hospitals, day care centers, hot-line centers, and prisons can add a great deal to the course. Internships can be much more valuable than field trips, even if students participate for just one or two hours a week. The extended experience gives students a much greater exposure to the complexities of medical situations.

Academic standards should be applied with the same degree of rigor as in any other part of the curriculum, even though evaluations cannot be based on knowing a correct answer. However, evaluations can include development of understanding of or the ability to deal with a particular problem. Case studies can help, as can evaluative instruments which require the identification of the underlying dilemma in complex decision making.

Teachers and administrators should be aware that any bioethics program will meet with some criticisms because of its somewhat innovative teaching approach and the sensitive nature of its subject material. A teacher would be wise to describe a new program carefully to colleagues and administrators, and to introduce it only if there is a consensus for acceptance. Institutes of bioethics, professional associations, and administrators could be helpful in making specific suggestions to a teacher whose program does not receive initial acceptance, or whose program does not fulfill the intended goals.

B. UNDERGRADUATE EDUCATION*

I. Existing Programs

Within the regular curriculum of undergraduate colleges one often finds courses in biology for nonbiology majors. These may include some passing attention to ethical or public policy issues. Similarly, introductory courses in ethics offered by departments of religion or philosophy may include a unit on "the biomedical revolution" or some specific issue, for instance, abortion. Full unit course offerings in biomedical ethics are becoming more common as a part of permanent curricula.

Undergraduate courses in bioethics tend to have one of two characteristic foci. Some are concerned with global issues such as population problems or ecology; these are characteristically approached from a scientific viewpoint. Another kind of course concentrates on the moral crises in the doctor-patient relationship (e.g. truth-telling, euthanasia); these usually are taught by philosophers or theologians. In all this many possibilities are left unexplored: the study of medical themes as they are expressed

*This section of the report was written primarily by David H. Smith, Associate Professor of Religious Studies, Indiana University, Bloomington.

in the arts and literature, the analyses of relationships among health professionals, the relationship between the medical professions and the public.

II. Goals

Undergraduate education is concerned with more than the development of professional skills or the acquisition of factual knowledge. Competencies may, and information certainly will, be acquired in a good college education, but more basic than either is the development of, first, a method for finding needed information and, second, the critical ability to understand, marshal, or evaluate an argument. Well-educated people know how to find out what they need to know and are able to assess the various conceptual schemes used to organize, interpret, explain, or evaluate facts.

This suggests that good courses in bioethics should avoid two dangers. First, they should not be concerned solely with solving practical problems. Second, they should not simply present relevant biological or scientific facts. One thing anyone concerned with this area can learn is that "the facts" change rapidly; today's "right solution" is tomorrow's dogma. Thus, undergraduate offerings in bioethics must have a *focus* beyond problem solving and popular biology and *upon questions of normative theory*. This should not justify use of biomedical problems as a pretext for teaching the unaltered clichés of one's own discipline, but it does imply that providing the facts or the "right answer" is, at best, insufficient. Preoccupation with the study of ethical and value *theory* is especially important on the undergraduate level.

III. Course Organization

It is important to try to cover diverse topics (such as abortion, etc.) as well as to present different normative theories (teleology vs. deontology). A straightforward approach which has worked well is to isolate two important types of ethical

theory and then to show how their users resolve specific normative issues. When successful the result is to introduce the student to a range of bioethical issues while giving him or her the
theoretical competence to criticize alternative assumptions and
arguments. Ideally, the student acquires the rudiments of a personal ethical theory. The theoretical diversity makes indoctri-
nation almost impossible; the use of multiple topics awakens
the student to new practical problems—or at least places familiar ones in a new light.

Such a course presents many problems, however. The attempt to cover a huge range of topics inevitably means that
some, if not all, are given short shrift. Thus, a promising varia-
tion of this type of course would be to select one topic (euthanasia, sterilization) or family of topics (death and dying, control
of reproduction) and cover it in more depth. The teacher could
then present a greater diversity of options on the level of normative theory as well as encourage detailed study of the interdisciplinary complexity of the topic. The alternative—presenting
only one theoretical viewpoint while surveying a diversity of
topics—might be very effective with advanced students of normative theories, but not on the introductory level.

IV. Teaching Formats

First, it is important to remember that although many undergraduates in this country have been anesthetized by media bom-
bardments depicting every possible bizarre (and not so bizarre)
human crisis, their own experience of life is often relatively
sheltered. They have probably not been physicians or researchers, experimental subjects, the parents of a defective
baby, or even touched by the death of a parent. If their reasoning about biomedical ethics is not to be artificial, therefore,
they must *experience* some of these things vicariously. This may
occur through use of audiovisual materials, visiting professionals
or patients, or literary works. The instructor's responsibility is
to make sure that this vicarious experiencing is not done to
shock, to indoctrinate, or to divert attention from the deepest
issues of the course; all these are real dangers. Nevertheless, a

course in biomedical ethics can bridge the gap between popular wisdom and academic criticism; it should be taught in a way that capitalizes on this opportunity.

Second, good courses in biomedical ethics will inevitably be *interdisciplinary* in one sense: the expertise of practicing physicians, academic biologists, attorneys, legislators, social scientists, and humanistic ethicists is relevant to almost any specific topic one might name. Thus, these courses provide a rare opportunity to get a college community talking to each other about things that matter—and to get it talking with members of a nonacademic community. A course must draw on—and it contributes to—various specialties.

Third, if students are to understand bioethics, they must *discuss* the course material. This is because bioethics material is rooted in practical problems, is interdisciplinary, and has some theoretical focus. It is hard to imagine a successful course which uses only a lecture format. Furthermore, this discussion must be *critical* yet *open*. Somehow a sense of the urgency of the issue and the students' obligations to express their views (however shocking) must be combined with the notions that no one's views are beyond criticism and that some answers are better than others. Some of us have discovered that tolerable discussion of this sort can be conducted in large classes, but obviously discussion is facilitated by small groups.

A fourth issue surrounds the use of "case method" teaching. The idea is adroitly to select (or, perhaps, to fabricate) a specific event or set of incidents which embodies at least one bioethical dilemma. Discussion of this case then can explore both a particular topic and a set of options in normative theory. This tactic has been used widely and is of prime importance to a successful bioethics course. However, the best way of integrating cases into a syllabus is not obvious. A course could begin with a case and be organized around the issues it opens; this procedure could be followed with every unit; or, a syllabus could be organized without reference to cases but regularly use them as pedagogical heuristic devices. In a more extreme vein, an entire course could be taught inductively, with each class session centered around case discussion, following the practice of law and business schools.

We do not intend finally to pronounce on the merits of these approaches, but will confine ourselves to three general remarks. First, extensive use of cases does help provide the kind of vicarious experience that seems desirable in most undergraduate situations. Second, use of a totally inductive case method runs the danger of failing to delineate general theoretical issues; unless one can assume that the students have, or will acquire through reading, a fairly high degree of sophistication, the result may be collapse into practical problem solving. Finally, there is obviously a relationship between the size and level of a class and the appropriate format. In very general terms, we think that the smaller and better a class is, the more useful case methods will be.

V. Administrative Structure

We think that the importance of the issues of bioethics requires the *development of regular course offerings* in all significant institutions of higher education. Extracurricular coverage does serve to stimulate interest, but its obvious inadequacies as a teaching mechanism are the very reason for the existence of formal curricula. "Experimental curriculum" coverage is not much better. These courses are often taught in a faculty member's "spare time"; they may reflect an avocation rather than a professional expertise; they may be taken for small amounts (or no) credit. They tend to titillate and provide an opportunity for airing opinions—rather than to educate. A regular course offering, sponsored by a department or program, in no way automatically solves any of these problems; it does provide an institutional mechanism through which they can be tackled, and it establishes clear accountability when the tackle is missed.

Second, our commitment to multiperspective or interdisciplinary work in bioethics does not lead us to conclude that undergraduate courses *need* be interdepartmental. Such an arrangement may be appropriate when new courses are introduced into the curriculum, and may be required over the long haul for a particular course in a given institution. But we worry about the lack of focus and continuity that may be involved, and suspect that course quality will be better sustained if responsibility finally rests with one faculty member, program, and/or department.

Third, we think that sound curricular development suggests that there be a correlation between the expertise of the teacher and the essence of the subject taught. Thus, fundamental responsibility for developing courses in bioethics should rest with those departments which are, in one way or another, concerned with normative questions. Broadly speaking, this means the humanities and social sciences, or at least departments such as philosophy and religion where ethics is usually taught.

Fourth, major institutions should move beyond a one course approach to this subject because a one semester (or quarter) course cannot *both* pursue several topics in depth *and* survey the range of topics in this field. If one course is designed as a survey, students should have further opportunities to pursue awakened interests. If, on the other hand, one course focuses on a particular topic (death and medical killing, experimentation on human subjects), then a vehicle for study of others should be provided. Then, too, it is important that value questions be studied from more than one perspective. While primary teaching responsibility may rest with ethicists, biomedicine also clearly raises social-scientific and aesthetic value questions. It is impossible and undesirable to isolate bioethics from its broader context. Development of a family of courses using varying methods and at differing levels of specialization can be facilitated through the creation of an interdisciplinary committee or program.

VI. Future Needs and Priorities

The greatest need at the undergraduate level is to encourage the development of courses in humanities and social science departments. Professionals in those areas need to be awakened to the possibilities of the field; they also need to be exposed to the biomedical realities. To this end some fellowships of variable length should be created to enable humanists and social scientists to prepare themselves for teaching and research in bioethics. The grantee should spend his residence in a setting where exposure to both the real workings of biomedicine and the reflection of other humanists and social scientists is accessible.

In addition, it is not too early to worry about the continued professional growth of those who have become interested in issues of bioethics over the past five years. New journals are probably unneeded, but the development of programs in professional societies, and of inter- and intradisciplinary conferences, will require continued subsidization.

C. MEDICAL SCHOOLS*

I. Existing Programs

Bioethics is becoming more significant in the medical curriculum and many schools now support faculty teaching in this area. As evidence, a 1974 Hastings Center survey of 107 American medical schools revealed that ninety-seven (91 percent) were teaching medical ethics in some form. Only six (6 percent) schools gave required courses, but forty-seven (44 percent) offered electives. The remainder incorporated medical ethics teaching into other courses or special lecture series. This paper will propose and discuss elements we believe should comprise an adequate program for teaching ethics in medical schools.

II. Goals

Of the four teaching goals described in Part One, the first three seem of particular importance in medical school programs: identifying moral issues, developing strategies for analyzing moral

*This section of the report was written primarily by Albert R. Jonsen, Associate Professor of Bioethics, Departments of Medicine and Pediatrics, School of Medicine, University of California at San Francisco; and Charles M. Culver, Associate Professor, Department of Psychiatry, Dartmouth Medical School.

problems, and relating moral principles to individual cases. These goals must be integrated with a broader one of medical education: the development of the physician's understanding of patients as individual sick people. This occurs less by formal instruction than by the example of experienced physicians and the atmosphere of medical education. However, a program in bioethics can provide the student with an important intellectual framework within which to understand the moral dimension of relationships with patients.

The third goal, that of relating moral principles, rules, and intuitions to specific cases, seems particularly suited to medical school bioethics teaching. It parallels the general structure of medical education in which general principles and ways of organizing data are first learned, then skill in applying this systematic knowledge to individual cases is developed by practice.

We believe teaching should not be construed as aiming to produce a physician who is in some way a more "moral" decision maker. Although doubtless doctors must sometimes make moral choices which they cannot easily transfer to patients or others, our aim is to train physicians who can create relationships with their patients in which moral decision making is shared. Our view of the appropriate doctor-patient relationship is similar to Robert M. Veatch's "contractual model," in which both doctor and patient understand that a certain class of medical decisions lies within the doctor's expertise, but that many decisions materially affecting the patient's life should be shared. Thus, we recommend that teaching focus as much on the process as on the moral content of the physician's behavior.

III. Curriculum Organization

A wide variety of courses and programs exists at present. They represent the ingenuity of their creators, local administrative support, faculty concern, and student interest. While encouraging such diversity and realizing that no single curricular organization is best, we suggest that certain forms are more suitable than others. Curricula should consist of courses designed to teach how to identify, define, argue, and work toward a resolution of ethical issues in medicine. Courses must have sufficient length and continuity to expose in an ordered way the lines of reasoning contributing to those activities. Naturally, a single lecture on some ethical aspect of a medical course's content might serve as an excellent appetizer. Required occasional lectures and readings in bioethics interspersed in the preclinical curriculum might provide a useful introduction to later discussions and seminars. However, simply interspersing ethics lectures among medical courses or offering lectures by diverse persons on various topics does not constitute a satisfactory program in ethics.

We believe that a basic introductory course should be offered and organized to allow extensive discussion. In some situations, this may be the only way to present ethics in the medical school. We hope that advanced elective seminars designed to pursue particular topics in depth can also be offered. In addition, occasional grand rounds, conferences, workshops, seminars, and consultations with housestaff provide opportunities to deal with specific ethical issues. It is particularly important to set up regular and structured opportunities for house officers and students in their clinical clerkships to discuss morally problematic cases. A regular clinical-ethical conference (strongly supported by the chief of service), which provides retrospective analysis of a difficult case, is very valuable, since, as most physicians agree, the clinical years and internship are the most formative in their medical education. None of these, however, substitute for a well-designed introductory course.

While it seems preferable that courses be offered as electives or as options among a range of required electives, they must carry academic credit. Finally, these courses should be taught at a reasonable time and place. This often requires considerable ingenuity, since there are numerous claims on the schedule of medical students.

IV. Teaching Formats

Only an intensive seminar format seems to permit adequate practice of the necessary skills in moral perception, reasoning, and problem-solving. Instructors should propose cases or moral problems, actively lead students through their analysis, and explore all opinions in an attempt to reveal underlying principles and assumptions. Role-playing of physician-patient interactions is often useful.

While we believe that a seminar format is nearly indispensable, it can be accompanied by various techniques, including readings, audiovisual presentations, and even occasional short lectures. Readings should be carefully designed clinical cases and short, well-focused background articles. We think students assigned too many articles often disregard them. Our preference for small seminars should not obscure their danger of becoming easily unfocused. Discussions should center on isolating accurate information and performing careful analysis.

In Part One of this report, course structures were divided into topical, thematic, or methodic; and thematically organized courses were said to be most useful in medical school teaching. Introducing themes with illustrative cases is frequently a desirable way to prepare students for subsequent more abstract discussion.

It seems appropriate that moral aspects of the individual doctor-patient relationship receive heavy attention in medical school teaching. However, proper treatment of the course's themes should not only consider individuals in medical situations but also stress the institutional and cultural frameworks that influence their actions. Clearly, certain social and historical forces influence and constrain the behaviors and choices of both doctor and patient.

V. Qualifications for Teaching

Before stating criteria for qualified instructors, two frequent problems must be noted. First, the wide interest in bioethical issues has prompted certain physicians, who are little acquainted with the discipline of ethics, and certain ethicists, unfamiliar with the art of medicine, to enter the field. It is more likely that the former will offer a course in ethics in medical schools. While such persons may become skilled in ethical analysis, it is possible that their personal moral concerns and their medical knowledge may produce an ethics course which is a display of problematic cases, well described medically, but poorly analyzed ethically. We think that since ethics is a proper academic discipline with a long tradition in Western thought, it should be taught by those acquainted with its methodology and history. The presence of highly motivated but poorly trained amateurs is detrimental both to medicine and to ethics.

Second, it is sometimes said that ethics is best taught not by an appointed professor but through students' association with many ethically sensitive medical practitioners. This is dubious for two reasons. (1) The character, emotions, and sensitivity of persons may be appreciated, absorbed, and imitated by such osmosis without students gaining any skill in analyzing moral problems, which is the proper work of ethics. (2) Medicine's moral problems are as complex as its technology; they are not analyzed by simple wisdom or solved by benign character. We believe that their consideration requires trained skill in ethical analysis and ample time for research and reflection.

The nature of bioethics teaching in a medical school setting calls for the cooperation of ethicists who know medicine and physicians familiar with ethics. Ethicists are trained to deal with ethical discourse in terms of the theory and history of their discipline. Physicians' clinical experience and scientific knowledge enables them to evoke the medical context vividly and sensitively. These distinct perspectives are necessary to an activity concerned with not only the medical profession's behavior, but the common good of professionals, patients, and the public.

Thus, we believe that ethics should be taught in medical schools by a medically knowledgeable ethicist along with an ethically conversant physician. Ethicists should ordinarily have an advanced academic degree in philosophy or theology, with concentration in philosophical or religious ethics. They should have some formal initiation to clinical medicine and continued involvement while teaching. Ethicists should hold a proper academic appointment in a significant department of the medical school and should be invited to serve on appropriate faculty committees. Hospital chaplains should not be appointed teachers of bioethics merely on account of their clerical status or training; they should, in addition, have the qualifications mentioned above, namely, academic training in philosophical and religious ethics at the masters or preferably at the doctoral level.

Research and publication in medical ethics also requires appropriate academic qualifications and experience. Careful and informed scholarly work should be expected to issue from the cooperative endeavors of trained ethicists and ethically knowledgeable physicians.

VI. Administrative Structure

It is impossible to designate a single most suitable place for bioethics within the administrative structure of the medical school. Institutions are too diverse, local needs too unique, and personal interests too variable. However, we suggest that in most cases the bioethics program should not be isolated but rather should be located within a respected and traditional department, such as medicine, pediatrics, or psychiatry. The importance of the program is manifested by its place in the medical school structure. It does seem advisable, however, that, wherever located, one member of the bioethics team should be clearly designated as academically and administratively responsible.

VII. Future Needs and Priorities

A number of medical school courses and programs are requesting support from private and public sources. Since the extent of that support is limited, we suggest priorities which might guide the deliberation of funding sources. These priorities are chosen on the principle that those programs should be ranked higher which promise broader impact on the teaching of bioethics as the discipline develops.

First priority should be given to programs which intend to develop a research capacity in addition to their teaching responsibilities. The nature of bioethics requires not only ethical reflection and philosophical analysis but the amassing of factual information in such areas as medical practice, experimental protocols, delivery of health care, and the financing of medical care and medical education. Like scientific research in medical schools, bioethical research should accompany the teaching program and result in publication. Since such teaching and research programs will be housed by relatively few institutions, they should be initiated in a few selected medical schools.

Second priority should be given to teaching programs which intend to develop curricula for teaching bioethics. This is currently an important need of the discipline. Certain bioethics programs should establish curriculum development projects which other institutions may then employ in their own programs.

Third priority should be given to programs which intend to develop cooperative endeavors between institutions, particularly between institutions of different sorts, such as medical schools and divinity schools, law schools, or philosophy departments. In such cases, there should be tangible evidence of cooperation beyond mere expressions of intent by interested parties.

Fourth priority should be given to programs that intend only to present courses, lecture series, or occasional conferences.

D. NURSING SCHOOLS*

I. Existing Programs

Nursing programs are a very significant place for teaching medical and biological ethics. In fact, the impetus for much

*This section of the report was written primarily by the members of the Commission who have had experience teaching in nursing programs: Robert M. Veatch, Albert Jonsen, Jane Raible, Charles Culver, and LeRoy Walters. Consultation with Mila Ann Aroskar, R.N., Ph.D., School of Nursing, State University of New York at Buffalo; Elsie L. Bandman, Ed.D., R.N., Graduate Program in Psychiatric Nursing, Hunter College; Jeanne Q. Benoliel, Nursing Care, School of Nursing, University of Washington; Ramona Cass, R.N., Emory University; Ann Davis, R.N., Ph.D., School of Nursing, University of California, San Francisco; Noel J. Chrisman, Ph.D., School of Nursing, University of Washington; Phyllis T. Coletta, R.N., Villanova University; Maria C. Phaneuf, Professor Emeritus, Wayne State University College of Nursing; Joseph R. Proulx, R.N., Ed.D., Associate Professor, School of Nursing, University of Maryland; and Dolores W. VanDervort, R.N., MSN, is gratefully acknowledged.

bioethics education comes from nurses who have entered the clinical setting. Our investigation of teaching in nursing schools, however, finds that it is in a very fluid state. Many bioethics courses offered jointly by schools in medical centers are well attended by nurses. While nursing schools show a tremendous amount of interest in ethical questions, the evolution of formal courses and programs of ethics teaching seems to be less developed than in undergraduate and medical schools. A substantial number of teachers either are teaching or preparing to teach a course in a nursing school. Many nursing students are also enrolled in courses in undergraduate institutions. Continuing education courses for professionals are heavily attended by nurses. Specialists are developing at both the undergraduate and graduate level of nursing education who, through their own particular expertise (as R.N.s with Ph.D.s in sociology or cultural anthropology, for example) support the study of the psychosocial needs and rights of the patient in the curriculum.

However, few have been supported in this effort to develop courses explicitly emphasizing bioethics. Most often, ethical questions tend to arise from specific cases or problems which may develop in the classroom or clinical setting. One objective of nursing education is to clarify the nature of the nurse's responsibility to make decisions about patient care and hospital policy making.

The current focus for most formal bioethical education for nurses tends to be the psychosocial dimension of death and dying and care of the acutely ill patient; such courses tend to appear at the graduate level. What we have not found is the degree of specialization in ethics teaching that has emerged over the past five years in other educational institutions. There are to our knowledge no instructors in nursing schools with a title "professor of ethics" or its equivalent. There are no formal "programs in ethics." There are a few opportunities for nursing students to take elective courses. Some are taught in conjunction with medical schools or philosophy departments. Even these seem to be primarily in baccalaureate programs. Students in associate degree and diploma programs which are not affiliated with a university or medical center seem to have a particular need for teaching opportunities and support. Most people teaching ethics in nursing schools are currently doing so as a secondary activity, while their primary responsibilities are either some other aspect of nursing education or some other dimension of ethics teaching outside the nursing context. The specialists who have an overview of the development of nursing ethics education have not yet emerged. There is some evidence that nursing ethics text writing and curriculum development is beginning. Generally ethics as an integral part of nursing education is a seriously overlooked area, one which deserves far greater attention than it has received.

II. Goals

While all the goals of bioethics teaching outlined in Part One of the report are significant for ethics teaching in nursing schools, nursing students find themselves in a unique situation. While they tend to be attuned to patients' personal and social needs and spend more time with them than physicians do, they are also traditionally socialized into a subordinate position in the health care team. Thus, they may perceive ethical problems in medical care—such as a patient's distress on not being told of his or her condition. They may be asked to inject the terminally ill with morphine in a dosage that could be meant to kill as well as relieve pain. Whatever ethical doubts they may have about these judgments, they may feel powerless to override the physician's decision that the patient should not be further informed. Yet nurses increasingly feel themselves liable morally and legally for patient care decisions. They may strive to overcome their feeling of moral powerlessness by increasing the weight assigned to their own ethical evaluations, but they thereby risk imposing their own values on the patient and family. Nonparticipation alone is not enough. Nurses must be able to take a moral position in a logically consistent manner congruent with more than a nodding acquaintance with ethics. Especially with the increased questioning of the nurse's role vis-á-vis the physician's, problems of power, authority, and conflict resolution, which have ethical implications, must be addressed.

Thus, ethics for nursing students is not just a once-removed or watered-down version of the ethics taught in medical school. Nurses are involved in unique dilemmas and conflicts where their values are inconsistent with both the patient's and the physician's. In addition to helping students to identify and define moral issues and to develop strategies for analyzing moral problems, bioethics teaching for nursing students must focus more specifically on developing plausible models for the nurse's role as ethical decision-maker in relation to those of the physician and patient. This goal is associated with the third general aim of bioethics teaching: relating moral principles to specific issues and cases in such a way that students will be able to take a conscientious stand independent of physician or patient evaluations. An example might be objecting to participating in an abortion or to stopping a respirator even though instructed to do so. On the other hand, nurses will sometimes find it more appropriate to yield to patient values even though those might conflict with their own, the physician's, and/or supervisory nursing personnel's values. No student should leave nursing school without having confronted those ethical dilemmas inherent in the nurse's role.

III. Teaching Formats and Curriculum Organization

Every health care professional student should be exposed to some systematic teaching about ethical problems. There are great opportunities for diverse teaching formats. Opportunities for discussion—especially of specific cases posing ethical dilemmas for the nurse—seem to us to be essential for any well-developed program. *Ad hoc* case discussion, however valuable, is not sufficient; there must be more structured opportunities to deal systematically with classical ethical themes. Other teaching formats, such as case conferences, grand rounds, weekend workshops, and intensive specializations, also provide valuable breadth. Ideally, nurses should be expected to take a basic course in ethical theory before taking a course specializing in medical ethics. We recognize, however, that time pressures may not permit this. Courses which simply survey a series of topics in bioethics will be less adequate if they do not provide opportunities to discuss basic underlying themes.

IV. Administrative Structure

Faculty members, individually and collectively, should be competent in both the clinical aspects of nursing and the discipline of ethics. Since virtually no nursing instructors have professional competence in both simultaneously, team teaching should be the norm for the foreseeable future. All members of a team should preferably have professional standing in one area and competent amateur standing in the other.

One of the most significant administrative problems in ethics teaching for nurses is the relationship the course ought to have to courses offered for other health care professions and those outside the health care area. Ethics in nursing schools cannot be taught with the same models and problems posed in a course for medical students. While topics will, for the most part, be the same, the perspective is different. The dilemma of nurses caring for the comatose and terminally ill patient will often be quite different from that of physicians or the patient's relatives. They may have to decide whether to override the physician's instructions. They may have to cope with demands of the patient and family that the physician never encounters in inpatient and ambulatory care settings. Thus, an effective course for nursing students should address itself to these unique problems. At the same time, a great deal is lost if nursing students are isolated in a medical ethics course in which enrollment is limited to nursing students. We feel that there is great value in the exchange of perspectives which takes place among students with different career objectives. In some institutions, this may mean mixing nursing students with medical and other health-care-profession students. In others, it may mean mixing them with undergraduates who may be future business executives, lawyers, or simply concerned health consumers. Such a course could have special sections where nursing students could discuss the problems affecting them especially. The interchange, however, is critical, and should be given emphasis in designing ethics courses in a nursing context.

V. Future Needs and Priorities

We have identified three areas that must be addressed in order to provide effective learning experiences during nursing education. While some materials specifically oriented to ethical issues for nurses are beginning to appear, there is still a desperate need for basic literature, curriculum materials, case studies, and audiovisual materials.

Second, since there are virtually no trained teachers with adequate skills in both clinical aspects of nursing and ethics training, opportunities for faculty development must be given especially high priority. The one fellowship program designed specifically to train nurses in ethics had 200 applicants for two fellowships. There are no organized opportunities for ethics instructors who teach nursing students to get clinical exposure from a nurse's perspective. At least one such program should be established, probably through a graduate level program in medical ethics which has already organized similar general clinical training.

Finally, while workshops and conferences for medical ethics teachers in other teaching settings have existed for several years, there are virtually no such opportunities for nursing ethics instructors. Although conferences and workshops must be seen as preliminary experiences which will lead to more permanent professional communication networks, such gatherings would be valuable for nursing ethics instructors. Funding in all three of these areas is virtually nonexistent and would produce exceptionally great returns.

E. NONMEDICAL PROFESSIONAL SCHOOLS*

I. Existing Programs

Recognizing the growing impact of biomedical sciences and the need for professional persons to be prepared to help their clients confront bioethical dilemmas, many professional schools now offer instruction in bioethics. Typical courses are "Genetics and Law," "Health and Human Rights," "The Physician and Society," and "Eugenics and Justice." In many universities such courses are offered in or open to students in schools of public health, nursing, law, and related fields.

Moreover, some schools now offer degree programs with a concentration in bioethics. The emergence of such programs suggests that new categories of professional persons may be established eventually.

II. Goals

Nonmedical professonal schools such as law, public policy, and theology have specific educational objectives, which may shape the goals of teaching bioethics: training for advocacy roles requires a different curriculum than training for counseling skills. Further, not all members of a profession will share the same depth of involvement in bioethical issues. The educational needs of those who choose a career focusing on bioethics (such as a ministry specializing in hospital chaplaincy) will differ from the needs of those who will encounter bioethical issues only sporadically in their work.

Nonetheless, all professional schools share certain educational goals which set the context for teaching. First, professional persons generally function as counselors, advocates, and policy-makers; thus professional schools share the goal of training per-

*This section of the report was written primarily by Karen Lebacqz, Assistant Professor of Christian Ethics, Pacific School of Religion, Berkeley, California.

sons to assume such roles. Second, professional schools provide socialization into a profession. As students assume greater responsibility in a profession, they may become more deeply involved in the issues encountered. Recognizing the importance of this involvement, many professional schools provide "field exposure"—direct experience in professional practice. Incorporating teaching bioethics into the process of socialization is an opportunity particularly appropriate to professional schools.

Within this context, the teaching of bioethics has four goals. The first goal is to help students learn to recognize and define moral issues arising in biomedical research or practice. For example, the minister called upon to counsel a distraught couple whose newborn child has a genetic anomaly must be equipped to recognize and identify the ethical dilemmas they face.

The minister or other professional must not only be able to distinguish those aspects of such a situation which are specifically bioethical dilemmas, but also have enough technical knowledge to explain options open to parents. A second general goal, therefore, is exposure of students to sufficient technical information and clinical settings so that they will be prepared to offer options to clients and to recognize additional areas for investigation.

Professional persons will be called upon to help their clients analyze moral issues or to advocate public policy for change in biomedical arenas. The third goal of teaching bioethics at the professional school level is therefore the development of strategies for analysis of moral issues. Professional schools must provide training in normative ethics. This goal is, of course, particularly important where professional persons choose to focus a career on bioethics.

The fourth goal is to help students develop skills for applying normative analysis to a variety of case situations.

As more students encounter bioethics in their undergraduate curricula, the teaching of bioethics in professional schools may require different structures and objectives. The shape of graduate professional education in bioethics will need periodic modification.

III. Curriculum Organization

For those who will not be focusing their careers on bioethical issues, a *thematic approach* is the most suitable. It will indicate general themes that recur in bioethical dilemmas, and alert the professional to the need for more in-depth analysis in specific problem situations.

Those who choose to focus their professional work in bioethics will need more *in-depth methodological analysis* as well as more exposure to a variety of topical issues. The thematic approach can be supplemented by advanced study in methodology and exposure to a wide variety of clinical settings.

Some professional schools may choose to maintain a curriculum reflective of the orientation of the school rather than broadly representative of all aspects of biomedical ethics. For example, a law school may confine its offerings in bioethics to those related specifically to the law. Such specificity is intended to ensure that a student will develop the particular skills needed for practice of a particular profession.

IV. Teaching Formats

To fulfill the goal of enabling professionals-in-training to encounter dilemmas that they will face in professional practice, a *case-study approach* may be the most effective format. In our experience, most professional students become impatient with lecture formats that do not allow them to apply their learning to case situations.

Discussion sessions related to *field experience* is a particularly appropriate context for teaching bioethics; and a field leader trained to recognize and help students approach bioethical issues is invaluable.

Since students at this level of education need to develop skills in normative analysis, instruction may *combine lecture with discussion*. However, since the objective is to make the normative analysis a working part of the student's professional skills, the focus should be on discussion and on teaching formats which enable students to utilize their knowledge.

V. Administrative Structure

In professional schools with a department of ethics (most seminaries), the most appropriate central focus for a curriculum in bioethics is in that department. However, courses taught in other departments ("Counseling the Dying," "Theological Perspectives on Pain") would certainly be considered an integral part of the total curriculum. Indeed, it is conceivable that the bioethics curriculum might be administered out of another department (such as theology).

In professional schools that do not have a department of ethics (most law schools), the program or curriculum in bioethics will tend to be administered out of whatever department develops the interest and/or funding. Thus a curriculum in bioethics may originate under the auspices of a department of jurisprudence or family law. However, it is preferable that the administering department be able to demonstrate considerable competence in analytic methodology, either through its internal staff or through arrangements with trained professionals from other schools or departments.

Persons in several departments may teach courses related to a bioethics curriculum utilizing their specialties ("Legal Aspects of Experimentation"), though these courses may not specifically focus on ethical analysis. Determination of appropriate titles for such courses (for example, whether they should be called "bioethics") lies within the jurisdiction of the professional school (and, to some extent, the professional societies to which its faculty belongs).

VI. Qualifications for Teaching

In general, we propose that the establishment of a program in bioethics and the designation of courses in "bioethics" are most appropriate when a trained ethicist is involved. Some professionals trained in other disciplines who have worked extensively in normative ethics will qualify as professional ethicists for this purpose. Determination of qualifications for teaching rests with the individual school.

Lawyers, theologians, and other professional persons not trained extensively in the discipline of ethics should be encouraged to teach courses within their spheres of competence which may be part of a bioethics curriculum.

The pattern of team or interdisciplinary teaching which is prevalent in many professional schools is probably best suited to the needs of most students. This approach reflects the wide range of persons involved in bioethical issues in their professional practice, and allows each professional person to use her or his competence to the fullest.

There is one special case in which the professional person is also a trained ethicist. In seminaries with a department of ethics, the professional most likely to deal with topics in bioethics will have extensive training in normative ethics, making it unnecessary to include another trained ethicist. In this case the team approach may be advisable to allow collaboration on medical or legal aspects of bioethical issues.

VII. Future Needs and Priorities

Priority should be given to those institutions which:

1. Develop interdisciplinary programs or curricula, in particular those which combine the orientation of the particular professional school with the disciplines of medicine and ethics;

2. Develop new professional specialties, for example, the Doctor of Ministry, with a focus in bioethics;

3. Combine a significant teaching component with research so that some wider impact on the community can be achieved;

4. Develop new curricular options—field exposure training situations, audiovisual tools for teaching bioethics, and so on.

F. CONTINUING PROFESSIONAL EDUCATION IN BIOETHICS OUTSIDE DEGREE PROGRAMS*

I. Existing Programs

Existing bioethical centers cannot meet the increasing demand for continuing education in bioethics for the professional in health care and in the humanities (whether academician, clinician, lawyer, or clergy). Most professionals seeking skills in bioethical reflection and decision making—especially the physician and nurse in private hospital practice—cannot or do not wish to enroll in long-term internships, sabbaticals, or in-degree programs. The demand upon the variety of short-term workshops and conferences increases annually as interest in bioethics grows. The development of *ad hoc* programs in hospitals and academic settings is evidence of the growing demand for such outside-degree continuing educational programs.

Some continuing education courses in bioethics offer credits. In general, however, enrollment seems to be only slightly affected by credits offered, because most persons seek such education to solve special problems which arise in their own professional lives (for example, to determine the proper decision-making mechanism in care for the high-risk neonate). Awareness that traditional value assumptions do not always fit developing problems can create practical dilemmas which bring many professionals to the proliferating workshops and conferences. One such dilemma is posed by the mental retardate of majority age who cannot obtain an abortion in a state which permits abortion because the retarded citizen is now "overprotected." Professionals do not want to become conversant in metaethics but to deal with immediate and practical concerns.

There is, however, a rapidly growing trend toward acquisition of continuing education credits annually as a requirement for continued state medical licensing. Many states have already passed

*This section of the report was written primarily by Jane A. Raible, Executive Director of the Northwest Institute of Ethics and the Life Sciences, Seattle, Washington.

such statutes requiring continuing education of physicians. More significantly, increasing numbers of medical specialty groups, such as the American Academy of Family Physicians, have passed requirements for continuing education annually as a condition of membership in that specialty. Many more specialties require CME (continuing medical education) for recertification in that specialty; an example is the American Board of Surgery. State nursing associations as well as specialists in medical records and pharmaceutical practice are also developing similar requirements. What constitutes such continuing education is loosely defined, and bioethical conferences/courses are a potential focus, provided they meet the specialties' own criteria for continuing education credit. Such a trend vastly influences increasing numbers of health care professionals to seek accredited continuing education courses sponsored by their specialty, by university extension, and by those bioethical centers which meet the specialties' criteria. The majority of these courses are not in-degree programs, although they carry continuing education credits.

Most often, courses available vary widely in style and format expressing the needs of the setting in which the courses are offered (medical schools, medicolegal symposia, high school biology teachers' conferences, nephrology technicians' workshops) and the skills of the faculty. Funds available, accessibility to academic and/or bioethical centers are all factors which affect the variability and scope of these proliferating bioethical programs. The variety contributes both to the vitality and disparate quality of the growing discipline. Thus, although much continuing education is conducted outside degree programs, it can, and increasingly the trend is that it does, carry the credit required by many professional groups, especially those in health care.

II. Problems

Problems of professional continuing education which especially affect nondegree (but often credit-bearing) offerings include:

1. *Limited course availability.* Adequate opportunities close to home do not exist in most regions.

2. *Time limitation.* Most professionals (local physicians, nurses, clergy) have limited time and money for long-term study away from home.

3. *Interdisciplinary study.* Much of the demand for courses emanates out of a specific hospital service/unit (for example, nurses in pediatrics) or a particular university department (for example, medical geneticists providing community counseling), or a specialty (for example, American Board of Internal Medicine). Such courses tend to reflect the values and concerns only of that service or department or specialty. The richness of interdisciplinary approaches to bioethical education is critical and often lost under such auspices.

4. *Pedagogical style.* Technologically oriented professionals who may have the greatest need for awareness of bioethical complexities often, through their own professional socialization process, expect to find "answers" to their dilemmas. It is difficult to communicate that no easily applicable "right" answers exist in bioethical issues. In fact, it is not easy to move beyond the specific case under discussion to an analysis of recurring issues.

5. *Faculty limitations.* The very variabilities in training and vision of faculty offering courses in bioethics contribute greatly to the creative variety of pedagogical styles but can also create the situation in which some instructors become side-tracked in fad issues, neglecting the larger dilemmas and broader application of themes. Such instructors are often forced to offer courses on their own time without department support.

6. *Motivation.* By definition, continuing education does not attract individuals able to devote much time to outside study although the degree to which many do outside work is indicative of their depth of interest. Most are working in full-time practices or jobs and such continuing education must be developed with that time limitation in mind.

7. *Professional limitations.* Some medical services and professions tend to be more open to reflection upon developing technology and its effect upon human beings and social policy while others are closed to such questioning either among colleagues or in interdisciplinary forum. Openness to such discussion also varies from institution to institution. Willingness to participate in interdisciplinary continuing education also varies with professions; for example, nurses are more receptive to such mixed learning situations than are most physicians.

III. Goals

Most often, professionals seeking opportunities for bioethical discussion and study desire an overview of the field. Their concerns arise out of a specific issue which confronts their daily professional life. Although the presently popular courses on death and dying may seem faddish, the interest they stimulate provides entry into the entire field. In reality, then, course goals most often focus upon highly specific dilemmas in which the professionals feel uncomfortable and seek strategies for decision making; for example, the neonatal intensive care unit or the physician whose patient manifests a genetic disorder which can affect profoundly the child-bearing risks of other distant family members. Yet such courses provide learning occasions which can be broadened to include identification and definition of recurring moral issues. But to move beyond the case specifics to relating general moral principles of the case to other bioethical dilemmas is a major triumph and greatly dependent upon the skill and philosophical knowledge of the faculty. The primary goal of outside degree professional continuing education is, then, decision making in a specific case. It is to be hoped that the skill of the instructor is adequate to the task of reaching the deeper goals of bioethical education as described in Part One.

Continuing education in bioethics is thus mostly *applied ethics*, ethical issues which arise out of specific situations. To the degree that the instructor is skilled in bioethics, that specific need can become the opening wedge into the wider field of applied ethics in biomedicine.

Additional goals for continuing education of professionals in outside-degree (but often credit-bearing) programs include:

1. Developing health care professionals with competent amateur status who are informed by more than the values attained through their professional socialization, institutional routines, personal assumptions, and "received values."

2. Understanding that no easy answer or paradigm exists in bioethical issues which can be learned once and applied forever without danger of ignoring the complexities of the issues and recognizing that bioethical education is a life-long professional process.

3. Focusing upon practical professional issues as entry into theories of ethics as applied to the life sciences.

4. Clarifying the impact and responsibility of professionals in health care and the humanities as leaders in the development of social policy within clinical and institutional settings as well as change agents in health care legislation.

5. Broadening the awareness of the diverse perspectives with which various professional groups and institutions view issues.

6. Assisting health care professionals to feel more adequate in their task of helping people in need, comfortable with their own responses and more aware of the variables in human needs, values and decision-making priorities.

IV. Teaching Formats

A great variety in format and style of education models exists in such courses, including:

A. Two-three day conference offered usually to a specific profession by the continuing education division of a university or profession—with or without credit

Pro

- Participants are highly motivated.

- If quantity of attendees reached is a goal, this format works.

- A setting is provided in which a broad overview of the field can whet appetites for more in-depth study later.

- More professionals are willing to participate in short-term courses (e.g. American Medical Association fact sheet on Continuing Medical Education April 1976).

Con

- The concentrated time span limits reading and assimilation.

- Participants may feel that they have "learned" that field.

- Large groups frustrate the need for discussion and lead to feeling that speakers have answers listeners can acquire.

- Personal agenda/problems triggered by topics cannot be met (especially in fields of death and genetics).

B. Five-ten week course in specific school setting

Pro

- In-depth discussions possible in such small groups.

- Interdisciplinary interchange is maximized unless format used is debate of advocate positions rather than true engagement of ideas.

- Ability to use varying skills, differing professional expertise and expertise of class members is maximized, i.e. collaborative learning.

Con

- When offered as part of a system or profession, co-opting/advocacy is a potential high risk.

- Style of teaching in specific institutions often precludes creativity and interdepartmental cooperation.

- Administrative overhead/criteria place value on enrollment and fees thus emphasizing large classes which reduce opportunity to exchange ideas/reflections.

C. Five-ten week course outside a school setting: (includes both professional credit and non-credit bearing courses)

Pro

- Institutional co-opting is eliminated and allows freer discussion and value evaluation.

- Freedom from established structure in size, format, meetings and professional vested interests is enhanced.

- Highly motivated individuals participate, especially when no credit or scholarships offered.

- Instructor must rely on ability and record rather than on tenure or safety within system.

- Ability to use varying skills, differing professional expertise and expertise of class members is maximized, i.e., collaborative learning.

Con

- Establishment of legitimacy of course is difficult outside the institution, although specialty groups seem open to granting professional credit when presented by well-known bioethical centers.

- Such classes become highly motivated yet self-selected groups which eliminate the rank and file of the professions.

- Advocacy positions are often presented rather than a forum.

- Regulation of quality of teacher/course is difficult.

D. One-night (afternoon) event

Pro	*Con*
• Issues and emotional responses are quickly surfaced which can open the entire field and encourage people into continuing education.	• Ability to develop skill in evaluating recurring issues is severely limited.

V. Curriculum Organization

The *ad hoc* nature in which so many conferences and courses develop suggests that it is fortunate if the class can be moved beyond the specific case or clinical dilemma to the evaluation of recurring moral issues. The format which initially entices people to enroll is one which is short in duration (two-day intensive conference or a five-seven week course) requires little outside work, and centers on topics of immediate concern rather than themes, such as genetic counseling, consent in clinical trials or rights of the dying patient.

Several administrative problems are critical. What incentives can be offered to encourage enrollment and outside study? Such enticements include offering "comp" time, courses on shift or credits through professional organizations. Courses which offer specialty continuing education credit create incentives and force the course provider to meet criteria of the specialty groups in order to grant credit for the course. These incentives force an accountability of the instructor for evaluation and quality.

The origin of the request for courses has its effect: a prime impetus for continuing education in bioethics arises in the nursing services, which often means that few physicians will attend. Location of the course carries weight, as those offered within a single hospital or a single service, for example, are limited in value perspective unless particular attention is paid to securing an interdisciplinary staff. Settings in which both the teaching staff and the enrollees reflect a variety of disciplines and professional value perspectives enrich the learning process. Additionally, interdisciplinary courses enhance the learning potential when class members' expertise is utilized by the faculty in a shared learning setting.

VI. Qualifications for Teaching

It seems obvious that persons qualified to teach courses in bioethics in the settings described should be professionals in either health care or one of the humanities (preferably ethics, philosophy, or theology) and that they have developed and *maintained* through ongoing personal education a competent amateur status in the related field. Legitimization and credibility of the faculty is rooted deeply in the sense of the class members that the faculty member is skilled not only in a profession such as social ethics, but also has developed and maintained by ongoing personal education an accurate perception of what it means to be a physician in the emergency room, for example, and the trends in that service.

VII. Future Needs and Priorities

The burden of on-going, in-service training and continuing education in bioethics for professionals in their work settings will fall upon individuals who are competent professionals in their own fields (for example, physicians who have skills in ethics and philosophy), and who have maintained competent amateur status in those related fields. Inasmuch as professionals (lawyer, physician, minister, nurse, social worker, academician, and legislator) are critical shapers of social health care policy, high priority must be given to their continuing needs throughout their professional lives.

The development of staff training programs for such teachers in their own professional settings is critical. Neither adequate teaching materials and training programs exist nor is there a clear delineation of goals for bioethics teaching for working professionals and evaluative tools for measuring course effectiveness. The development of high quality courses to train competent amateurs and teaching materials for use in their own settings is of highest priority so that professionals, after they receive basic bioethics education in their professional schools, can (1) maintain those important skills throughout their professional lives as biomedical advances change the nature of the ethical dilemmas they face and (2) serve as teachers of bioethics in their own clinical/professional settings.

It is the nature of developing biomedical advances that no answers can be learned for bioethical dilemmas and thus such education must be seen as a life-long process. Thus there is, together with firm programs in professional schools with adequately trained faculty, the additional critical and growing need to provide the opportunities, staff, and teaching tools for an education process in bioethical reflection and decision making which continues throughout one's career.

G. ADULT EDUCATION*

Participants in adult bioethics education programs have two special characteristics. On the one hand, they constitute an audience of incredible diversity, since in a sense everyone is a potential student. On the other hand, they are unlikely to be seeking credentials and are more likely to be seeking practical assistance in the resolution of everyday problems and conflicts associated with bioethical issues.

Hence adult bioethics education is designed to serve the lay person as individual citizen, voter, peer informant, patient, and "biomedical actor" rather than the professional-in-training as college student, physician, lawyer, nurse, philosopher, or biologist. It tends to be an attempt to impart "tools for living" rather than professional skills. It needs to be very diverse and flexible, with an *ad hoc* element, since the interests of the audience and the topicality of the issues can seldom be predicted.

*This section of the report was written by Michael Henry, Associate for Education, Institute of Society, Ethics and the Life Sciences, with the assistance of Jane Raible, Ruth Kolman, and Karen Lebacqz.

I. Existing Programs

Present activities in adult bioethics education are of two types. The first general type is that of community-oriented courses and activities, occurring most commonly as college extension courses, community college courses, adult education courses, issue-specific education programs (widow support groups, parents of mentally retarded, etc.), and community health center activities. Although it is difficult to generalize about the quality and quantity of these courses, it is probably fair to say that they include some of the best and some of the worst educational experiences in the bioethics area.

The second general type of activity is mass media attempts to highlight bioethics issues, including television talk shows, news presentations, medically oriented regular programs and special documentaries, as well as radio programs, and newspaper and magazine articles. The mass media always simplify, sometimes sensationalize, and occasionally reinforce misconceptions on bioethics issues. However, mass media presentations also occasionally serve to set norms and expectations for technological change, for medical progress, and for the mechanisms of medical decision making, and clearly can serve as vehicles to arouse interest. While we might hope that adult bioethics education is undertaken as part of carefully designed and sensitively implemented courses and activities, it is obvious that the mass media presently serve as a major source of educational experiences in this area and cannot be ignored.

II. Goals

The major goal of adult bioethics education is to increase the individual decision maker's consciousness of the ethical issues in biology and medicine, through exposure to a range of topics, themes, and alternative approaches. The individual can, it is hoped, thereby identify and define moral issues in biomedical science more easily, and develop and apply a personal framework for evaluating alternatives and relating moral principles to specific issues and cases. Intuitive responses can then be analyzed with respect to their value base, and individual problems and conflicts can be discussed and approached sensibly and rationally. An additional important goal is to enable the individual to sharpen the perception of his or her ability to deal with the existing health care system as a consumer.

III. Teaching Formats

For such goals to be achieved, a one-time lecture clearly cannot serve as the format for a bioethics educational experience for adults. In order for students to be exposed to even a minimal range of topics and alternative approaches, the best format is one based on small amounts of time over a longer period, rather than intensive short courses or sessions, particularly since most participants in an adult education program are likely to be totally unfamiliar with the issues. Also, in order to develop an individual framework for relating moral principles to specific issues and cases, the student needs time. *Ad hoc* media presentations are not likely to satisfy this requirement; nor are most of the current piecemeal adult education courses available. The best educational experience for the lay adult in this area is most likely to be a gradual, developmental approach.

IV. Curriculum Organization

The curriculum for an adult education course must strike a delicate balance somewhere between, at one end, sensationalism and overconcentration on specific cases, and, at the other end, excessive probing into the philosophical and ethical dilemmas so that individual interest in practical conflict resolution is lost. There is clearly a need to spark interest in the issues and topics, and maintain it with good treatment of specifics, but excessive use of case studies can prevent the equivalent concentration on general ethical issues. Yet, while a thematic approach may be best in many bioethics courses, adult education classes should concentrate more on topics with less emphasis on themes. The courses may consist of treatment of a series of topics of current interest, with an underlying theme, such as the individual as decision maker, being brought out from time to time.

The choice of topics can be dictated by the participants' likely interests. For example, every adult will probably have to deal, implicitly or explicitly, with such issues as cadavers, health insurance, patients' rights, individual responsibility for health (for example, smoking), and the tolerance of mental and physical diversity. Many adults will also need to deal with such issues as living wills, organ transplantation, genetic counseling, malpractice, informed consent, and terminating treatment. These topics will each attract the strong interest of some participants, while affording the teacher an opportunity to bring out underlying moral themes and value issues and demonstrate alternative approaches.

V. Qualifications for Teaching

The question of who teaches an adult bioethics education course will depend a great deal on the participants and curriculum. While a variety of people might be best to demonstrate a variety of perspectives, such an arrangement makes it more difficult to draw out a unifying theme. It would perhaps be preferable to have one teacher address many topics, assuming her or she had the required minimal competence in both ethics and biomedical sciences, so that a wide range of different topics can be covered at the same time that underlying themes are drawn out. It is worth noting, however, that a variety of teachers acts as a "drawing card" for a course.

If there is any one teaching skill which is to be valued above others in this area, it is discussion leadership. Students will need to work through their own philosophies, in order to develop problem-solving skills which are based on their own value systems and moral frameworks. The skillful discussion leader could well be much more important to the success of a course in this area than the highly skilled lecturer, particularly since a topical approach requires constant updating. Another valuable teaching skill is the ability to identify and build on whatever relevant professional knowledge and skills and/or personal experiences the participants may bring to the course. This would be particularly helpful in cases where the participants have skills or experience that the teacher lacks.

VI. Future Needs and Priorities

The area of adult bioethics education is so poorly developed that the needs constitute a list of considerable length. Three areas of need stand out, however, as of higher priority than others. First, there is the need to identify and train potential teachers who could serve as community leaders for adult education programs. Perhaps the most convenient source of such trainees is those community residents who have previously acquired relevant skills—nurses, clergy, physicians, biology teachers, retired professionals, for example—and who could serve as teachers of community courses in bioethics with a minimal amount of retraining.

Second, the need for minimal facilities for courses in the community has to be addressed. Existing community centers, high schools, churches, and other accepted community institutions could be used to a greater extent by incorporation of adult education bioethics courses, community health center activities and other bioethics educational programs.

Third, there is a great need to develop appropriate mass media materials at the adult level for bioethics education. Most of the current programs on television are rudimentary and generally inappropriate, as are most of the pieces used currently on radio and in newspapers and magazines. There is little variety and many of the producers of such materials are constrained by inexperience in this area, insufficient time, and/or overly inhibiting budgets. Also many mass media materials are not easily transferred to adult education courses, which means a waste of potential teaching aids.

Thus, the most immediate needs for funding in this area are for identifying and retraining potential local teachers, and attracting them (and eventually their students) to courses and other bioethics educational activities. If interest is stimulated among potential teachers by the availability of support for training, facilities and materials will follow. In the meantime, however, at the state and federal level there is an urgent need for funding to be channeled toward the development of appropriate mass media materials. Support is needed for a series of public television documentaries, and for free-lance writers and journalists to attend workshops and devote time to article and story development in this area. We need teachers and materials addressing bioethical issues with excitement, clarity, and simplicity, but without sensationalizing and without glossing over the very deep dilemmas which individuals are being forced to resolve, without help, in this area every day.

H. PH.D. AND M.A. PROGRAMS IN BIOETHICS*

I. Existing Programs

Graduate level training in the field of bioethics is offered by a small but growing number of universities. As of mid-1975 about ten master's or doctoral programs were available in the United States. In terms of the number of graduates produced, however, no large-scale programs exist.

Current programs are generally located within university departments of philosophy or religious studies. Two distinct program models can be identified. In the first a graduate student has the option of custom-building a program which includes bioethics as a major emphasis. The second type of program is structured in advance by a university department and offers an integrated series of courses which provide a concentration and subspecialization in the field of bioethics. In both models the graduate degree awarded is an M.A. or Ph.D. in

*This section of the report was written primarily by LeRoy Walters, Ph.D., Director of the Center for Bioethics of the Joseph and Rose Kennedy Institute for the Study of Human Reproduction and Bioethics, Georgetown University, Washington, D.C. We wish to thank James Childress and Tom L. Beauchamp for their helpful comments on an earlier draft of this section.

some field of the humanities. However, since bioethics includes subject matter from numerous disciplines, graduate programs in the field generally draw upon extradepartmental educational resources—from other departments, professional schools, or university-affiliated research institutes.

Perhaps because of the interdisciplinary character of bioethics, it has been proposed by some that a third model be created, namely, a graduate program which would culminate in an M.A. or Ph.D. in bioethics rather than in a traditional discipline. Supporters of this proposal note that significant social and scientific developments frequently result in the creation of entirely new fields, for example, sociology or biochemistry. Critics of the proposal reply that interdisciplinary graduate programs sometimes lack focus and that, given the predominance of the departmental structure at most universities, such programs may be doomed to failure. We believe that if existing departments are sufficiently flexible to incorporate the type of program outlined below, there is no current need for special graduate departments, divisions, or schools of bioethics. In the future, however, the development of the field and/or changing social priorities may at some point allow, or even require, the creation of new academic structures for graduate education in bioethics.

II. Goals

The primary aim of Ph.D. programs in bioethics is to train future teachers and researchers. This goal requires an integrated program of coursework, supervised teaching, and direct observation and experience. The program should also provide the student with basic bibliographical skills. Potential locations for Ph.D. graduates include university departments of philosophy or religious studies, medical schools, divinity schools, schools of public health, government agencies, and research institutes in bioethics or related fields.

In contrast, the goal of the M.A.-level programs in bioethics is to provide a basic education in bioethics for professionals whose primary expertise is in another area. The graduates will have a better understanding of the central issues of bioethics and will be able to contribute fresh perspectives to their own professional fields and also become involved in the teaching of bioethics. Among the professional groups which may be most interested in enrolling in M.A. programs are physicians, lawyers, policy makers, and university or high school teachers.

III. Curriculum Organization and Teaching Formats

The curriculum proposed for graduate programs in bioethics depends in part upon one's conception of the scope of the field and in part upon one's philosophy of graduate education. What follows is a suggested curriculum outline which presupposes a broad conception of the field and which affirms the value of supervised teaching and directed experience within a graduate program. (It is a composite of elements from several existing or projected graduate-level programs in bioethics.)

The "ethics" half of bioethics points to the humanities component of the field—most notably, the formal study of ethics, as that study has been pursued by moral philosophers and religious ethicists. This component should include an introduction to the history of ethics and intensive study of both ethical theory and applied ethics. The recurrence of traditional ethical themes and the emergence of possible new themes in the literature of bioethics should also be noted.

Two additional areas of humanistic inquiry go beyond the boundaries of ethics but are useful components. The first is the philosophy of mind, which investigates questions like the relationship between the mind and brain and the concept of "person." The second is that broad and somewhat amorphous area called the "philosophy of medicine." This division of the philosophy of science concentrates on philosophical presuppositions of the biomedical fields and explores such fundamental concepts as "health," "life," "purpose," "organism," and "evolution."

The "bio" half of bioethics represents the biomedical component of the field. No graduate program in bioethics would be complete without a comprehensive state-of-the-discipline review of current and anticipated developments in biology, medicine, and psychology. This synoptic "Introduction to the Biomedical Fields" requires the careful coordination of data from numerous basic-science disciplines and clinical fields. It should provide the most important information about each area as well as a method for updating one's knowledge in the future.

Two other subject-matter areas are not so clearly linked to the term "bioethics" but serve to complement the components outlined above. These are:

1. A social science approach to the biomedical fields through studying the history, sociology, anthropology, and economics of biomedical research and health care.

2. A public-policy approach to the biomedical fields through the fields of law and policy studies.

Teaching formats in graduate-level programs should be adapted to the subject matter and to the numbers and educational needs of graduate students. A lecture and discussion model will probably be most adequate for the state-of-the-discipline survey; the seminar format seems better suited to the analysis of issues in the philosophy of medicine. Media presentations and case studies can complement the lecture and seminar formats. Term papers and examinations should be directed toward encouraging the student to integrate the admittedly disparate materials included in the graduate program.

There will probably be a significant amount of curricular overlap between the first year of the Ph.D. program and the M.A. program. Professionals in the M.A. program can be excused from courses in which they are already experts and can instead help to teach such courses. For example, a lawyer enrolled in an M.A. program in bioethics might be one of the teachers in a course entitled "Law and the Life Sciences."

Supervised experience is a second program element which can be shared by both M.A. and Ph.D. students. Within this internship or clerkship program an attempt should be made to provide students with direct exposure to clinical care, research involving human subjects, basic laboratory research, hospital administration, and the formulation of public policy in the biomedical fields. The one-year M.A. program will probably allow only two months for supervised experience. Up to six months of the Ph.D. program can profitably be devoted to the internship and clerkship programs.

Three curricular elements will be unique to the Ph.D. program. The second-year program of coursework for Ph.D. students will normally include advanced seminars and reading courses in areas of the student's primary interest. Each Ph.D. student should also be involved in a program of supervised teaching at the undergraduate level. Finally, the writing of a dissertation will serve to integrate the various elements of the student's graduate program and to provide in-depth studies of particular issues in a field where few such studies have as yet been done.

IV. Qualifications for Teaching

Since long-term competence in multiple fields is a virtual impossibility, it seems likely that specialists in a variety of related fields will need to be a permanent part of graduate programs in bioethics. Specifically, faculty members with graduate or professional degrees in the following specialties will be required: philosophical and/or religious ethics; the philosophy of biology or medicine; the history of medicine; the sociology and anthropology of medicine; medical economics; law; biology; psychology; and medicine. An ideal qualification for all of these persons would be one year of graduate training or its equivalent in one of the other fields included in the program.

As specialists in bioethics emerge from graduate programs, they will become important bridges to second-generation Ph.D. programs in bioethics. Many will no doubt function as coordinators of such programs.

V. Future Needs and Priorities

The first priority in the near future should be the development of excellent graduate programs in bioethics at several universities. If possible, each university should have ready access to a medical school. The various graduate programs in bioethics should be encouraged to develop distinctive approaches and teaching methods, so that each program may profit from the experience of the others.

Extra-university funding will probably be required for start-up administrative and faculty costs of such programs. Such support could be granted on the basis of five-year external support and a commitment by each recipient university to continue the program for at least ten years following the initial grant support period.

A second priority is fellowship support or training grants for able persons willing to undertake graduate study in the field of bioethics. This support could be subdivided into two categories. One-year fellowships would allow professionals to enroll in M.A. programs; graduates would then return to their home institutions to take part in bioethics teaching. Three- or four-year fellowships would enable a first generation of specialists to gain Ph.D.-level training in bioethics and to become teachers of the next generation of students in the field.

PART THREE

Priorities for Teaching Bioethics

In Part One of this report we described four general goals to be pursued in teaching bioethics: (1) developing skills in identifying and defining moral issues in biology and medicine; (2) developing strategies and analyzing moral problems; (3) relating moral principles to specific issues and cases; and (4) training a group for careers in bioethics.

Students ranging from elementary and high school to professional and graduate school ought to learn at least some of these skills. Part Two presented the scope of bioethics teaching at eight educational levels. Only an integrated approach to bioethics teaching will adequately meet the needs of so varied a student body. Any overly narrow view of the priorities for teaching, such as limiting teaching emphasis to physicians and other medical professionals, must be resisted.

Yet not all efforts are equally important. Priorities must be established in any field of study, especially at the relatively early stages of its evolution. Part Three of this report addresses some of these emphases in programming, teacher training, and funding, seen from the perspective of three years of investigation of the teaching of bioethics.

These priorities are determined in view of the goals on which we all agree. These goals can be attained, we believe, by starting with the development of certain resource centers from which persons, ideas, information, activities, and materials will emanate. These resources are necessary to begin the more extensive and more varied teaching activities. Our principle of priority, then, is to concentrate effort and funds on those endeavors

61

which presently promise the most intensive development of the resources necessary for the gradual achievement of the widespread, effective and superior teaching of bioethics on an ongoing basis. The objective is to generate a seeding effect beginning with a small number of high-quality programs in order to assure quality and competency. We use this as our principle for ordering the way we think the field should develop. Of course, we are not implying that broader, more diversified teaching efforts are, in the long run, any less significant. Without them the goals we have outlined could not be achieved. We are not ranking priorities in order of importance, but rather in order of recommended chronological development. We are thus proposing what we think is a sensible progression for the development of bioethics teaching.

Priorities

1. *We consider it critically important that a few first-rate, comprehensive, research-oriented programs become firmly established.* These should be programs which will contribute to building the reputation and legitimacy of the field. Such programs should combine solid research with varied course and other educational offerings. Because the subject matter affects the general public, it should be taught so that people can use the teaching in making decisions about their own lives. But we cannot do this without research centers. While in general all academic departments in all institutions need not have research components, it is essential that in any given field at least some programs be solidly committed to the development of ideas and materials. Research and resource centers should be designed to meet varying needs and objectives of those teaching in the field. Criteria for evaluating such centers include:

   a. Geographical diversity.

   b. Distinctive orientation and specific subject expertise.

   c. Interdisciplinary orientation.

   d. Capacity and commitment for consulting and research as well as local teaching concerns.

   e. Ability to teach in several modes such as college and professional school courses, conferences, post-doctoral fellowships, workshops, etc.

Some of these centers may be within university settings, but others may exist outside that framework. When such research-oriented teaching programs are firmly established, then other, more directly teaching-oriented efforts have a foundation upon which to build. Such programs will also be a major source of materials—scholarly literature, texts, audiovisual materials, etc.—which can be used in other teaching efforts.

2. A second kind of effort which should receive special priority is *teacher development which has a "seeding effect," that is, which generates its own momentum for the evolution of teaching in the field.* Among the programs currently serving this function are graduate programs training teachers in bioethics and teaching workshops and fellowship programs designed to add necessary interdisciplinary skills to those already trained in one relevant professional discipline.

Since an interdisciplinary specialization such as bioethics will require training in more than one basic discipline, most teachers in the field will be required to obtain what we have called "competent amateur" status in the related disciplines. "Seeding" programs which can bring a teacher into the status of a competent amateur in the subsidiary disciplines deserve highest priority. Of course, different levels of teaching will require different amounts of cross-disciplinary exposure. For university and professional school teachers with doctoral level training in their basic field of competence, the equivalent of at least one year of intensive training in the subsidiary discipline is strongly recommended as an ideal. For those teaching at the elementary and secondary level and for those in adult and other nonformal academic programs, at least a university level course, a summer session training program, or the equivalent will be essential. Fellowships to support training of teachers are seriously needed.

In general we believe that the primary emphasis should be placed on courses taught by those with adequate skills in both the scientific and philosophical areas. At the university level this means that bioethics courses taught under that name should be taught by someone who has had adequate training in both the sciences and ethics (by attaining at least competent amateur standing in the field outside his or her primary training). In some cases it will be preferable for the courses to be taught on an interdisciplinary basis, by a team with both professional and competent amateur skills. At the level of training other health science professionals, interdisciplinary training seems to us to be essential. Professional competency in both ethics and the medical sciences must be present on an equal footing. Any training program which will provide adequate skills at the various levels deserves special priority.

After considerable discussion within the commission about the desirability of setting standards of certification for competency in bioethics teaching, we concluded that *at this point we do not recommend any formal body for certification.* Clearly the standards for a qualified teacher will vary depending upon the teaching level. They will also vary depending upon the resources available by other members of the teaching team. We do hold that anyone teaching in the field should continue to meet the standards and certification (formal or informal) for his or her parent professional field. Thus a philosopher should be presumed to meet the standards of a professional philosopher; a clinician, those of his or her field necessary for a teaching appointment. We do not, however, recommend that efforts be made to set up a professional organization of bioethics or a certifying committee for subspecialization in bioethics.

3. *For purposes of teaching of bioethics, courses which have specific ethics content should be given priority.* Courses taught under other rubrics such as "technology and society" or "social problems in medicine" have a significant role in the educational process. We think it is important that the difference be recognized and that for bioethics or medical ethics courses priority should be given to courses that are oriented toward the explicit nature of ethics in the teaching. The exact nature of that content will vary, depending upon the level of the teaching. Formal metaethical analysis is appropriate for a graduate program in bioethics, but more general exploration of conflicts in values and principles may be more fitting in a high school. At all levels, however, the commitment for bioethics teaching must be to explore explicitly ethical problems, not simply psychological and sociological ones.

In contrast, teaching efforts which fail to provide a minimum exposure for the intended purpose should be given low priority.

While the one-shot lecture or special program has a legitimate function—to arouse interest in a field or educate on a very specific problem—it seems to us to be generally inadequate and to imbue the subject matter with a sense of faddishness or transiency. Educational efforts such as guest lecturers, lecture series, and conferences deserve low priority unless they lead to further educational efforts of greater depth or unless they are sufficient in themselves to accomplish a specific educational objective. They might arouse medical student interest in an on-going series of courses or might serve to inform a community group interested in, say, the ethics of a specific health care problem in the community. Unless they can be defined on these grounds, however, they seem to us to be of secondary educational importance.

4. Another area which we feel deserves high priority is the *preparation of good materials for mass media and audiovisual use in the classroom.* A few such materials are currently available, but the selection is very limited and often the high-quality materials have to be used in somewhat inappropriate fashion. The production of a basic core collection of film and other mass media materials would be particularly valuable at this point in the development of the field.

5. While we stress that bioethics education must reach all levels from the young student to the professional with years of experience, *in general we think it is crucial to introduce the subject early, whatever the education level.* For example, while medical ethics education of the physician must include exposure throughout his clinical education, we consider it particularly important that conscious exposure be given as early as possible. Ideally, medical ethics should be part of the standard premedical curriculum. The student should be capable of the rudiments of disciplined thinking in medical ethics just as he or she acquires competency in the basic sciences. This early exposure has the added advantage of developing a framework for medical ethical thinking in a context which is not exclusively professional. The student has an opportunity to see the thought patterns not only of physicians and future physicians, but of future lawyers, business executives, and members of

other occupational groups. That kind of interoccupational educational exposure we consider to be particularly valuable, and deserves high priority.

6. *In order to maximize impact, funders should consider giving special priority to funding training and pilot programs in institutions where there is an explicit pledge to incorporate programs within the institutions' ongoing budget commitment in the future.* Thus there should be confidence that the teacher will have a continuing opportunity to make use of the training once it is received.

While funding priorities are closely related to general priorities for bioethics teaching development, they are not necessarily synonymous. Certain areas which we consider to be of high importance have had particular difficulty in receiving adequate funding. Secondary teacher training is one example. Another is the opportunity for those with primary specialization in ethics (philosophical or theological) to obtain competent amateur standing in the basic and clinical sciences. To this end one-year fellowships for humanists to spend time in clinical and research settings receiving formal training would be particularly valuable. The production of mass media materials is another area with particular funding needs. On the other hand, a number of pilot programs in the development of medical school ethics teaching have a demonstrated track record in being able to procure funds.

Ideals and Realities

While this report has discussed a variety of problems in the teaching of bioethics, and has put forth some ideal priorities, it would be remiss not to point out the larger context in which the teaching of bioethics takes place. That context may usefully be divided into two categories, the economic and the educational.

1. *Economic context.* At every educational level economic pressures are impinging deeply on the quality and direction of American education. Declining enrollments in primary schools and cutbacks in government funds for medical schools

are obvious examples. While those intent on introducing bioethics into a curriculum may well recognize that a systematic, solid, and ongoing program represents the wisest and most serious approach, they may count themselves lucky if they are able to find funds for even a short lecture series. Moreover, as a strategy to promote interest in bioethics, a brief lecture series may well have a valuable place as an introduction, as an occasion for locating potential supporters, and as a way of demonstrating to a reluctant administration that serious local interest in the field and the issues exists. In a context of economic scarcity, compromises will have to be made.

A few guidelines for making such compromises can be suggested. First, if bioethics must be introduced into an institution in far less than optimal ways, even that process should consciously be seen as only a first step; and plans, however tentative, for the next steps should be devised. Second, even if the first step is inadequate in terms of an ideal, it should be implemented as well as possible. Even a three-part evening lecture series done on a shoestring budget can be done well if care is taken in the selection of speakers, the format and the physical setting. Third, poverty can sometimes be survived. In most institutions it is still possible to organize informal study groups, for faculty members to invite other faculty members and students to their homes for discussion, and to organize faculty seminars or luncheons. If interest cannot be created in the absence of money, then money will not by itself create that interest. Of course, an unusual degree of dedication, private spending, and a willingness to sustain voluntary efforts over a long period of time are required.

Another increasingly serious economic problem is continuing programs or courses once started. Many institutions have, in effect, said that those intent on introducing bioethics into the curriculum are free to do so if they can find outside funding. In many instances this has been successfully accomplished. However, funds from private foundations are usually in the form of short-term grants with a stipulation that permanent support cannot be expected. The task then confronting the faculty member who has gained that development support is, at the end of the grant, to convince the institution to continue the program with its own resources. It is a delicate moment, made all the more poignant and painful by the fact that gaining permanent support may have little or nothing to do with the quality of the program. Many institutions, forced into retrenchment, have simply declared that no new permanent courses or programs may be introduced. There may well be no happy solution in that situation. The most that might be suggested would be a strong effort at the beginning of an outside grant to gain some minimal commitment on the part of an institution that an attempt will be made to incorporate the course or program into the permanent curriculum at the end of the initial grant period. These commitments may not, in practice, be of great solidity but they are worth trying to gain in any case. That the outside funding agency may require some such commitment as the condition for providing the grant can often provide a degree of useful leverage in that respect.

2. *Educational context.* In addition to economic problems, the current structure and ethos of many institutions presents additional problems. Despite much lip-service paid to interdisciplinary courses and programs, their actual fate is often determined by a range of well-known traditional structures and attitudes. One need only mention the usual problems of trying to organize courses which cut across the conventional departmental lines, of trying to convince unenthusiastic departmental chairmen or faculty committees of the value of courses which break with the standard departmental offerings, and of the hazards (particularly for young, untenured faculty members) of teaching and publishing in nontraditional areas.

Fortunately, at least at present, bioethics has a few advantages. Some money is available because of the interest of some private foundations and governmental agencies in the field. Funding can be a persuasive consideration even in the face of what otherwise might be hostility or suspicion. Student response to courses and programs in bioethics is often strong and enthusiastic. In universities which use a gross head-counting method of determining which courses are worth support, bioethics frequently does very well. This by no means proves that bioethics is a worthier subject for teaching than, say, Greek or medieval philosophy; it is only a fact of the times.

Yet this fact carries some long-term hazards. Like everything "new," bioethics can be subject to faddishness. At present, the strong media and public interest in medicine, the sometimes sensational quality of many of the problems in bioethics, give the entire field of bioethics a strong, outside boost. But how long will that last, and how soon will the public turn its interest to other problems? A course or program which, explicitly or implicitly, depends only upon public interest and popularity is destined for a letdown. Even more critically, if the issues are genuinely serious and difficult, as we believe they are, then an almost imperative first step in any course or program is to remove the faddish qualities of the topics and motivate students to serious work. The issues themselves deserve nothing less. Yet that puts matters on the highest plane. Even in terms of the gross self-interest of those concerned with the future of bioethics, nothing less than a convincing demonstration of the solidity of the field and the seriousness of its practitioners will suffice for its long-term survival.

Bioethics is a new field. It has yet to prove its intellectual value in any long-term sense, and it has yet to show that it can be as helpful and illuminating to students as any of the other myriad choices they may make in their educational process. We believe it can and will prove itself. But that will require a sustained and high level of work, a total seriousness on the part of those who work and teach in the field, and the willingness of those trying to advance the teaching of bioethics to be continually self-critical.

Over the past decade the teaching of medical and biological ethics has grown very rapidly. We see no reason for that trend to be reversed. What was adequate as an experimental effort five years ago, however, is no longer adequate today. If the field is to be taken seriously as a major area for learning, it must have maximum breadth. But it must also have solidity and depth. Only with careful attention to the development of systematic teaching and teacher training efforts will medical and biological ethics continue its growth into a significant interdisciplinary teaching field.

BIBLIOGRAPHY

Annas, George J. "Law and Medicine: Myths and Realities in the Medical School Classroom." *American Journal of Law and Medicine* 1 (Fall 1975), 195-208.

Babbie, Earl R. *Science and Morality in Medicine: A Survey of Medical Educators.* Berkeley: University of California Press, 1970.

Banks, Sam A., and Vastyan, E. A. "Humanistic Studies in Medical Education." *Journal of Medical Education* 48 (March 1973), 248-57.

Bennett, Glin. "Whole-Person Medicine and Psychiatry for Medical Students." *The Lancet*, March 29, 1976, pp. 623-26.

Blomquist, Clarence. "The Teaching of Medical Ethics in Sweden." *Journal of Medical Ethics* 1 (July 1975), 96-98.

Bluestone, Naomi R. "Teaching of Ethics in Schools of Public Health." *American Journal of Public Health* 66 (May 1976), 478-79.

Branson, Roy. "The Scope of Bioethics: Individual and Social." In *Ethics and Health Policy.* Ed. by Robert M. Veatch and Roy Branson. Cambridge, Mass.: Ballinger Publishing Company, 1976, pp. 5-16.

Brody, Howard. "Integrating Ethics into the Medical Curriculum: One School's Progress Report." *Michigan Medicine*, February 1975, pp. 111-17.

_____. "Teaching Medical Ethics: Future Challenges." *Journal of the American Medical Association* 229 (July 8, 1974), 177-79.

Callahan, Daniel. "Bioethics as a Discipline." *Hastings Center Studies* 1 (No. 1, 1973), 66-73.

_____. "The Emergence of Bioethics." In *Science, Ethics and Medicine.* Ed. by H. Tristram Engelhardt, Jr. and Daniel Callahan. Hastings-on-Hudson, N.Y.: Institute of Society, Ethics and the Life Sciences, 1976, pp. x-xxvi.

Churchill, L. R. "Ethos and Ethics in Medical Education." *North Carolina Medical Journal* 36 (January 1975), 31-33.

Clouser, K. Danner. "Humanities and the Medical School: A Sketched Rationale and Description." *British Journal of Medical Education* 5 (1971), 226-31.

————. "Medical Ethics: Some Uses, Abuses, and Limitations." *New England Journal of Medicine* 293 (August 21, 1975), 384-87.

————. *Philosophy and Medicine: The Clinical Management of a Mixed Marriage.* Philadelphia, Pa.: Society for Health and Human Values, 1975.

Cooper, John A. D. "Medical Education and the Quality of Care." *Journal of Medical Education* 51 (May 1976), 363-64.

Falk, Leslie, et al. "Human Values and Medical Education from the Perspective of Health Care Delivery." *Journal of Medical Education* 48 (February 1973), 152-57.

Ferrara, James L. M. "Medical Students: Future Physicians or Organic Mechanics?" *The Pharos* 39 (April 1976), 62-63.

Fox, Renée C. "Training for Uncertainty." In *The Student-Physician.* Ed. by Robert K. Merton, George G. Reader, and Patricia L. Kendall. Cambridge, Mass.: Harvard University Press, 1957, pp. 207-41.

Galletti, P. W. "Medical Ethics: How Much Can Be Taught?" *Rhode Island Medical Journal* 58 (February 1975), 39-40.

Gorovitz, Samuel. *Medical Ethics Film Review Project.* College Park: The University of Maryland, The Council for Philosophical Studies, 1974.

————. "Teaching Medical Ethics: A Report on One Approach." July 1973. (Available without charge from Moral Problems in Medicine Project, Dept. of Philosophy, Case Western Reserve University, Cleveland, Ohio 44106.)

Jones, J. S. P., and Metcalfe, D. H. H. "The Teaching of Medical Ethics in the Nottingham Medical School." *Journal of Medical Ethics* 2 (June 1976), 83-86.

Lief, Harold I., and Fox, Renée C. "Training for 'Detached Concern' in Medical Students." In *Psychological Basis of Medical Practice.* Ed. by Harold I. Lief, Victor F. Lief, and Nina R. Lief. New York: Harper & Row, 1963, pp. 12-35.

Pellegrino, Edmund. "Educating the Humanist Physician." *Journal of the American Medical Association* 227 (March 18, 1974), 1288-94.

————. "Medical Ethics, Education, and the Physician's Image." *Journal of the American Medical Association* 235 (March 8, 1976), 1043-44.

Risse, Guenter B. "The Role of Medical History in The Education of the 'Humanist' Physician: A Reevaluation." *Journal of Medical Education* 50 (May 1975), 458-65.

Society for Health and Human Values. *Institute on Human Values in Medicine*. Philadelphia: Society for Health and Human Values, 1974.

Veatch, Robert M., and Clouser, K. Danner. "New Mix in the Medical Curriculum." *Prism* 1 (November 1973), 62-66.

_____, and Fenner, Diane. "The Teaching of Medical Ethics in the United States of America." *Journal of Medical Ethics* 1 (July 1975), 99-103.

_____, and Gaylin, Willard. "Teaching Medical Ethics: An Experimental Program." *Journal of Medical Education* 47 (October 1972), 779-85.

_____, Gaylin, Willard; and Morgan, Councilman, eds. *The Teaching of Medical Ethics*. Hastings-on-Hudson, N.Y.: Institute of Society, Ethics and the Life Sciences, 1973.

_____, and Sollitto, Sharmon. "Medical Ethics Teaching: Report of a National Medical School Survey." *Journal of the American Medical Association* 235 (March 8, 1976), 1030-33.

Webb, Nancy, and Linn, Margaret W. "Value Change During the First Year of Training: A Comparison of Medical, Nursing, and Social Work Students." *Journal of Medical Education* 51 (May 1976), 427-28.